AF443524

INTEGRATION OF HEALTH TELEMATICS INTO MEDICAL PRACTICE

Studies in Health Technology and Informatics

Editors

Jens Pihlkjaer Christensen (EC, Luxembourg); Arie Hasman (The Netherlands);
Larry Hunter (USA); Ilias Iakovidis (EC, Belgium); Zoi Kolitsi (Greece);
Olivier Le Dour (EC, Belgium); Antonio Pedotti (Italy); Otto Rienhoff (Germany);
Francis H. Roger France (Belgium); Niels Rossing (Denmark); Niilo Saranummi (Finland);
Elliot R. Siegel (USA); Petra Wilson (EC, Belgium)

Volume 97

Recently published in this series

Vol. 96. B. Blobel and P. Pharow (Eds.), Advanced Health Telematics and Telemedicine – The Magdeburg Expert Summit Textbook

Vol. 95. R. Baud, M. Fieschi, P. Le Beux and P. Ruch (Eds.), The New Navigators: from Professionals to Patients – Proceedings of MIE2003

Vol. 94. J.D. Westwood, H.M. Hoffman, G.T. Mogel, R. Phillips, R.A. Robb and D. Stredney (Eds.), Medicine Meets Virtual Reality 11

Vol. 93. F.H. Roger France, A. Hasman, E. De Clercq and G. De Moor (Eds.), E-Health in Belgium and in the Netherlands

Vol. 92. S. Krishna, E.A. Balas and S.A. Boren (Eds.), Information Technology Business Models for Quality Health Care: An EU/US Dialogue

Vol. 91. Th.B. Grivas (Ed.), Research into Spinal Deformities 4

Vol. 90. G. Surján, R. Engelbrecht and P. McNair (Eds.), Health Data in the Information Society

Vol. 89. B. Blobel, Analysis, Design and Implementation for Secure and Interoperable Distributed Health Information Systems

Vol. 88. A. Tanguy and B. Peuchot (Eds.), Research into Spinal Deformities 3

Vol. 87. F. Mennerat (Ed.), Electronic Health Records and Communication for Better Health Care

Vol. 86. F.H. Roger-France, I. Mertens, M.-C. Closon and J. Hofdijk (Eds.), Case Mix: Global Views, Local Actions

Vol. 85. J.D. Westwood, H.M. Miller Hoffman, R.A. Robb and D. Stredney (Eds.), Medicine Meets Virtual Reality 02/10

Vol. 84. V.L. Patel, R. Rogers and R. Haux (Eds.), MEDINFO 2001

Vol. 83. B. Heller, M. Löffler, M. Musen and M. Stefanelli (Eds.), Computer-Based Support for Clinical Guidelines and Protocols

Vol. 82. Z. Kolitsi (Ed.), Towards a European Framework for Education and Training in Medical Physics and Biomedical Engineering

Vol. 81. J.D. Westwood, H.M. Hoffman, G.T. Mogel, D. Stredney and R.A. Robb (Eds.), Medicine Meets Virtual Reality 2001

Vol. 80. R.G. Bushko, Future of Health Technology

Vol. 79. A. Marsh, L. Grandinetti and T. Kauranne (Eds.), Advanced Infrastructures for Future Healthcare

Vol. 78. T. Paiva and T. Penzel (Eds.), European Neurological Network

Vol. 77. A. Hasman, B. Blobel, J. Dudeck, R. Engelbrecht, G. Gell and H.-U. Prokosch (Eds.), Medical Infobahn for Europe

ISSN 0926-9630

Integration of Health Telematics into Medical Practice

Edited by

M. Nerlich

Department of Trauma Surgery, University of Regensburg Medical Center, Regensburg, Germany

and

U. Schaechinger

Department of Trauma Surgery, University of Regensburg Medical Center, Regensburg, Germany

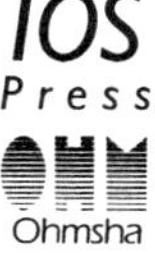

IOS
Press

Ohmsha

Amsterdam • Berlin • Oxford • Tokyo • Washington, DC

ISBN 1 58603 375 1 (IOS Press)
ISBN 4 274 90619 1 C3047 (Ohmsha)
Library of Congress Control Number: 2003110989

Publisher
IOS Press
Nieuwe Hemweg 6B
1013 BG Amsterdam
The Netherlands
fax: +31 20 620 3419
e-mail: order@iospress.nl

Distributor in the UK and Ireland
IOS Press/Lavis Marketing
73 Lime Walk
Headington
Oxford OX3 7AD
England
fax: +44 1865 75 0079

Distributor in the USA and Canada
IOS Press, Inc.
5795-G Burke Centre Parkway
Burke, VA 22015
USA
fax: +1 703 323 3668
e-mail: iosbooks@iospress.com

Distributor in Japan
Ohmsha, Ltd.
3-1 Kanda Nishiki-cho
Chiyoda-ku, Tokyo 101-8460
Japan
fax: +81 3 3233 2426

LEGAL NOTICE
The publisher is not responsible for the use which might be made of the following information.

PRINTED IN THE NETHERLANDS

Preface

In September 2002, telemedicine experts from all over the world gathered in Regensburg, Germany to join the **7th International Conference on the Medical Aspects of Telemedicine** with the topic **Implementation of Health Telematics into Medical Practice**. This conference was hosted by the Department of Trauma Surgery of the University of Regensburg, the German Society for Health Telematics and the **International Society for Telemedicine.**

During this conference, a unique exchange of research results took place, involving participants from 46 countries and 5 continents. All major topics of current telemedicine applications and research activities were addressed and an exchange of experiences in almost all fields of telemedicine took place during this 4 day conference. This so-called Regensburg telemedicine conference was probably one of the most important events of the international telemedicine scene. In order to preserve some of the many very interesting topics, we are publishing this book, which addresses very different subjects from research to practice and from medicine to information technology and medical informatics issues.

In most of the European countries, the United States, Canada, Japan and Australia, telemedicine is already helping to keep the health care systems under control, in terms of cost savings and quality assurance. This is reflected by significant funding from the governments of many of these countries, which are more than ever under huge pressure to keep the health care system alive. However, telemedicine has not yet reached mainstream medicine. There is only limited interest among scientists to address the issue of the impact of telemedicine on the current practice of medicine. Proper outcomes research on the effectiveness of telemedical applications would strongly establish the implementation of telemedicine in current medical practice. This is what makes this publication so valid.

Our goal is to keep up the good work, to make telemedicine more attractive than ever, use it as much as possible to improve delivery of health care and help us focus on the ethical basis of medicine: to serve the patient – as an individual and as part of our society – and that is the human aspect of modern technology.

The Editors

Acknowledgements

It was a great honor for us to host the **7th International Conference on the Medical Aspects of Telemedicine.**

We would like to thank all members of the scientific committee who actively contributed to the success of the conference as well as all participants who gathered for this telemedicine event.

Furthermore, the realization of the conference and this book would not have been possible without the support of some organizations, especially:

- the German Federal Ministry of Health;
- the Bavarian State Ministry of Labour and Social Welfare, Family Affairs and Women;
- the Deutsche Forschungsgemeinschaft DFG.

Special thanks to the individuals who worked on this volume:

- Helga Lautenschlager, Department of Trauma Surgery, University of Regensburg;
- Dr. Ekkehard Hundt and Mrs. Carry Koolbergen, IOS Press, Amsterdam, The Netherlands.

The Editors

Contents

Preface v

Acknowledgements vi

A Telemedicine Guideline for the Practice of Teleconsultation 1
Patrick Asbach and Michael Nerlich

Medical Telematics in Disaster Response 15
Thomas Benner, Ulrich Schaechinger and Michael Nerlich

Architecture and Tools for Open, Interoperable and Portable EHRs 25
Bernd Blobel

Telemedicine in Extreme Environments: Analogs for Space Flight 35
Charles R. Doarn

Development of a Robotic Navigation and Fracture Fixation System 43
*Bernd Fuechtmeier, Stefan Egersdoerfer, Georg Tuma, Gareth J. Monkman
and Michael Nerlich*

A Readiness Model for Telehealth: Is it Possible to Pre-determine How Prepared
Communities are to Implement Telehealth? 51
*Penny Jennett, Joanna Bates, Theresa Healy, Kendall Ho, Arminee Kazanjian,
Robert Woollard, Andora Jackson and Susan Haydt*

An Automated Diagnostic System for Tubular Carcinoma of the Breast – An Overview
of Approach and Considerations 57
F. Joel W.-M. Leong and James O'D. McGee

Data Analysis Now and Then: Significant Changes in Approaches and Results 73
Markus T.J. Mohr and Heinz Redl

Software Agents in Surgery: An Update 79
Markus T.J. Mohr

Technologies for Haptic Systems in Telemedicine 83
*Gareth J. Monkman, Holger Boese, Helmut Ermert, Dagmar Klein, Herbert Freimuth,
Michael Baumann, Stefan Egersdoerfer, Otto T. Bruhns, Alexander Meier and
Kashif Raja*

Cybercare NDMS: An Improved Strategy for Biodefense Using Information
Technologies 95
Joseph M. Rosen, Eliot Grigg, Susan Mc Grath, Scott Lillibridge and C. Everett Koop

A Communication-Theory Based View on Telemedical Communication 115
Thomas Schall, Wolfgang Roeckelein, Markus T.J. Mohr, Joerg Kampshoff,
Tim Lange and Michael Nerlich

Implementation of TeleCare Services: Benefit Assessment and Organisational Models 131
Karl A. Stroetmann, Veli N. Stroetmann and Chris Westerteicher

LifeGuard – Recording, Evaluation and Wireless Transmission of Medical Data 143
Bastian Arndt, Robert Krangemann, Markus Niklaus and Helmut Ulrich

NOAH – A Mobile Emergency Care System 147
Ulrich Schaechinger, Wolfgang Roeckelein, Alexander Perk, Patrick Asbach and
Michael Nerlich

Author Index 159

A Telemedicine Guideline for the Practice of Teleconsultation

PATRICK ASBACH, MICHAEL NERLICH

Department of Trauma Surgery, University of Regensburg,
Franz-Josef-Strauss Allee 11, 93053 Regensburg, Germany

Abstract. To establish a guideline for the use of teleconsultation, which is one of the most important applications in telemedicine beeing perfomed very frequently in daily medical practice in almost any field of medicine. Evidence: The recommendations are based on expert knowledge, because of the lack of evidence based data in the telemedical scientific literature. In addition, scientific articles of the highest level of evidence available published between 1970 and 1999 were reviewed.

Developement and consensus process: A guideline draft was prepared using the attributes of clinical practice guidelines developed by the Institute of Medicine (IOM) of the National Academy of Sciences. This draft was reviewed by telemedicine experts and the content of the guideline was approved by 100% group consensus in 5 meetings held between 1997 and 2000 by a panel of members of the Subproject 4 Group of the Global Health Care Application Project of the G8 countries.

Conclusions: The guideline gives recommendations on all aspects of teleconsultation in any field of medicine and will be updated regularly implementing new evidence

Introduction

The role of teleconsultation as a key element of telemedicine is continuously raising with the advances in medical and technological knowledge. Teleconsultation bridges the distance between health care professionals, significantly affecting the delivery of health care. It can transfer expert knowledge and direct treatment advice to underserved areas [1,2], and gives people access to a high level of health care without geographic restrictions [3]. It facilitates early decision making for disposition of a medical case [4], can serve as a triage tool [5] and be used for teaching purposes [6]. Teleconsultation can cut costs [4,7], as it has proven to be cost efficient [8,9,10,11] and time saving [12]. It speeds up the process of health care delivery [2,13] and improves patient and physician satisfaction [14,15,16,17]. Therefore it is an important tool to work with in order to solve a number of the currently most demanding problems in health care. Teleconsultation is used in almost any field of medicine including surgery [6,16,18], cardiology [7], pathology [2,19,20], dermatology [5,8,21], ophthalmology [9,22], neurology [23], neurosurgery [10], trauma surgery [4], orthopaedics [10,24], psychiatry [1], ENT [25], nuclear medicine [26], gynaecology [3], pediatrics [17] and neonatology [11]. Teleconsultation has very significant impact, especially in those fields of medicine that are on the increase and therefore are economically important, eg. diabetes [27], trauma [28] or wound care [29]. Although teleconsultation is in use in various settings in nearly every field of medical care, a generic guideline for practicing teleconsultation has to our knowledge not yet been published.

Background

To promote the development of a global information society, the governments of the G8 countries selected several pilot projects of international collaboration. Among those, the Global Healthcare Applications Projects (GHAP) set the objective to improve quality and cost-efficiency of healthcare delivery through the use of telematic tools. The main objective of subproject 4 (SP4) was to enable an international concerted action on collaboration in telemedicine. Science based methodology and expert clinical judgement, based on a three year collaboration of the G8 GHAP SP4 expert group, were used to develop specific statements on teleconsultation [30].

Objective

This paper is intended to provide a general approach to teleconsultation which is internationally viable. Based on the definition of consultation a generic definition of teleconsultation is given and the benefits and problems of teleconsultation are discussed. The purpose of this paper is to present a generic guideline for teleconsultation which is based on best-evidence synthesis.

This document provides a guideline for establishing policies and procedures to promote safe, high quality application of teleconsultation technology to the practice of medicine.

Guideline Development Process

Science based methodology and expert clinical judgement were used to develop specific statements on teleconsultation. Extensive literature searches were conducted, the databases searched include Medline, CINAHL, HealthSTAR, and ABI/Inform. Critical reviews were used to evaluate empirical evidence and significant outcomes. The quality of research evidence was evaluated using the criteria developed by the United States Agency for Healthcare Research and Quality:

I: systematic review or meta-analysis of multiple, well-designed controlled studies
II: at least one well-designed experimental study
III: well-designed, quasi-experimental studies such as non-randomised controlled, single group, pre-post, cohort, time series, or matched case-controlled studies
IV: well-designed non-experimental studies, such as comparative and correlational descriptive and case studies
V: case reports and clinical examples
VI: opinions of expert committees and other respected authorities

The recommendations are primarily based on expert knowledge, because the scientific literature was incomplete or inconsistent. Therefore the recommendations reflect the professional judgement of panel members and consultants. The guideline reflects the state of knowledge current at the time of publication. Given the inevitable changes in the state of scientific information and technology, periodic review, updating, and revision will be done.

Consensus Methods/Nominal Group Process

Consensus was obtained through peer review of drafts of the guideline and pilot review with intended users. Experts in various aspects of teleconsultation reviewed and commented on an early draft of the guideline, using as a framework for their evaluation the attributes of clinical practice guidelines developed by the Institute of Medicine (IOM) of the National Academy of Sciences [31]. Pilot review of a later draft was done with physicians, nurses, and others involved in teleconsultation at several clinical sites. They reviewed and commented on the clarity, clinical applicability, flexibility, resources or training needed to implement the guideline, and cost implications.

Key Guideline Recommendations

The intention of this draft is to provide a general approach to teleconsultation, which is generic enough to give interested health care professionals all over the world guidance in adopting the use of teleconsultation.

> *Definition: Teleconsultation is the consultation of one (or more) distant health care professional(s) by a locally present health care professional about a patient's case, diagnosis and treatment using telecommunication and information technology to bridge the spatial distance between the two (or more) participants.*

This definition identifies the communication partners as health care professionals who are legally legitimised to act as such in their place.

It is explicitly stated that this

> *communicational interaction takes place during the treatment process of a patient that requires either expertise that is not present at the place where the patient is or a second opinion of another expert in a difficult case.*

Furthermore it defines technological devices like telephone, videoconferencing tools and the internet as means to bridge the spatial distance between the health care professionals who are participating in the teleconsultation. Teleconsultation is very similar to a regular consultation. The health care professional conducting the treatment has to introduce the patient's case to a distant expert using the technological means chosen. Teleconsultation can be considered as one of the most common applications of telemedicine.

Benefits of teleconsultation: Teleconsultation can provide more accurate and accessible medical information anywhere and anytime, can improve quality of diagnoses and treatment through the access of expertise, can give the patient a higher level of confidence for the health care professional who performs the treatment [32] and therefore improve health care quality significantly.

Problems regarding teleconsultation: The degree of validation and the level of evidence in teleconsultation is low. Whether teleconsultation is superior to face to face consultation and where it is appropriate to be used remains to be determined. Evidence based or generally accepted guidelines for teleconsultation are currently not available.

STRUCTURAL ASPECTS OF TELECONSULTATION

Communicational Interaction and Organizational Integration

In certain situations teleconsultation is a viable and speedy alternative to the conventional postal way of sending information to consult expertise which is not locally available.

> *In a situation with the need of consultation of a medical expert, it has to be decided wheather the necessary expertise is localy available or not. If so, an "on-site" consultation can take place, if not, a teleconsultation should be performed (after the patient gave his consent).*

Teleconsultation is a communicative act by definition.

> *Teleconsultation consists of the communicational interaction of two (or more) health care professionals.*

The one who initiates the consultation has the intention to get information on the further treatment of a patient. He expects his addressee to be able to provide such a statement. For this reason he supplies the expert with a description of the case – eventually with diagnostic material to provide the best possible basis for a judgement. In return, he gets the answer of the expert – if the case description allowed a statement [33].

This process raises the question of the integration into everyday health care [4,34]. A few aspects of integration into everyday health care which apply generally can be identified:

> *1. Access: Every health care professional entitled to use the system has to have easy access.*
> *2. Ease of use: Since health care professionals neither are nor need to be experts in communication technology, the system has to be easy to use [34].*
> *3. Ease of contact: A list of the specialists to consult including the information how to contact them, must be available.*
> *4. Policy: The institution running the teleconsultation system should hand out a policy regarding teleconsultation [34,35]. It has to be compliant with local, national and international laws that are applicable. The teleconsultation policy must be announced.*

The guiding principle in organizing a teleconsultation should be adhere to the traditional way of organizing a health care consultation in the context of telemedicine. This will avoid disruption of the local health care system and preserve satisfactory relationship between the local health care providers.

For the elements "ease of use" and "policy" a clear definition of the workflow for conducting a teleconsultation can be identified. It should be a non-misleading ordered step-by-step description of the necessary tasks to fulfil in order to perform an efficient, policy-compliant, and legally acceptable teleconsultation. The following are the applicable steps outlining the generic workflow:

1. Search of an available expert to contact.
2. Decision on the medium to use; the local professional has to have access to the medium as well as the consultant.

3. Medium-specific preparation of the case description and request.
4. If the selected medium allows transmission of diagnostic material, the decision if diagnostic material should be transmitted, has to be made.
5. If diagnostic material should be transmitted, it has to be prepared, i.e. digitalized or imported into the case description.
6. If the medium allows synchronous consultation, the decision, if synchronous consultation should be done, has to be made.
7. If synchronous consultation has been chosen, the connection can be established and the consultational dialog can be held, eventually with parallel transmission of the diagnostic material.
8. If asynchronous consultation has been chosen, the response behaviour of the consultant must be agreed upon. In the case of frequent teleconsultation, a mutual agreement on this topic should be achieved.
9. In case of asynchronous consultation, the request, evenually including the diagnostic material, must be transmitted.
10. In case of asynchronous consultation, the reply must be retransmitted according to the negotiated response behaviour. This can be done by using a different medium, if negotiated. The described workflow can be visualized as an algorithmic diagram (Figure 1).

Technological Applications

A restriction on the technology that has to be used for teleconsultation can not be made, since all over the world multiple technological solutions have been used and are still in use to overcome the distance in non-local consultation in health care.

Communication Technologies: This list provides a basis to compare technological solutions against each other, it is not intended to evaluate ease of use and organizational integration of each technological solution.

The following features comprise the set to compare technological solutions for teleconsultation against each other concerning the capability:

> *1. to conduct synchronous ("on-line") consultation.*
> *2. to conduct asynchronous ("off-line") consultation.*
> *3. to transmit digital material.*
> *4. to standardize the technology for the use in health care.*
> *5. to compare availability of experts in a global setting.*
> *6. to verify the identity of the consultant instantly.*
> *7. to preserve the patients rights and privacy.*
> *8. to provide the means for the necessary documentation of the teleconsultation.*

The most commonly used media are telephone, videoconferencing and the internet platform (standard internet technology like e-mail, FTP (file transmission protocol), and the use of tools for the World Wide Web) and others. With the advance of internet technology various new tools can be expected, which will go far beyond the use of standard internet tools.

Figure 1. Teleconsultation Workflow

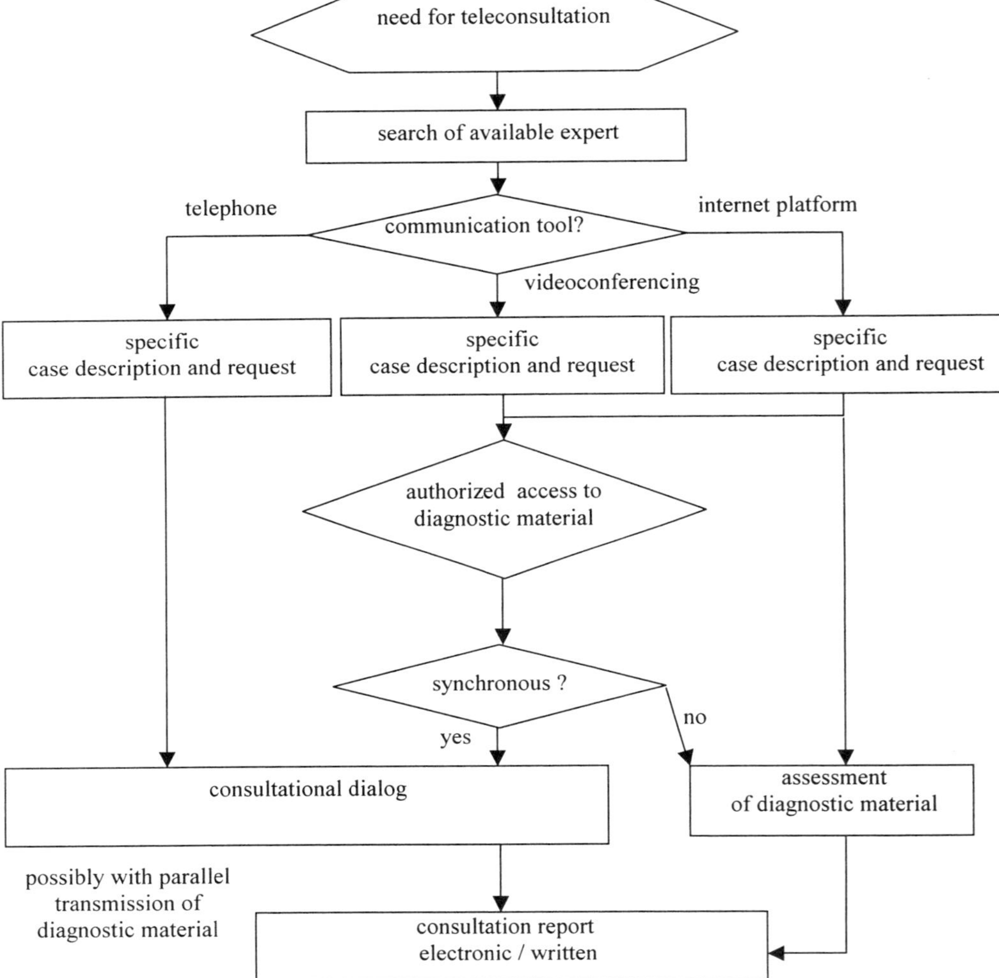

Synchronous communication: This feature describes, whether the technical solution enables the users to communicate in an on-line real-time dialog [4].

Asynchronous communication: In comparison to synchronous communication, asynchronous communication implies that the user´s statements are not given on-line, but rather that there is a time difference between a request and the following reply [4].

Transmission of diagnostic material: A central feature for the decision on a teleconsultation system is the question, if it is capable of transmitting diagnostic material.

Standardization: Protocols and standards are needed to guide the definition, acquisition, transmission, presentation, interpretation, multimedia storage, maintenance, and subsequent access and use of medical data.

Global availability: The feature of global availability describes the probability that a given expert independent of his place of residence has access to a technological basis for teleconsultation.

Verification of the partners identity: Although the verification of the partners expertise is mainly a matter of trust, the verification of his identity is an important feature of teleconsultation. From the legal standpoint it is absolutely necessary that the identity of the consultant is clear and unequivocal.

Patient's rights and privacy: Another essential feature of technology for teleconsultation is the way to preserve the patient's rights and privacy [35]. This means that the patient's informed consent about the teleconsultation can be communicated and his identity needs not to be revealed [32].

Inherent documentation: The matter of inherent documentation addresses the ease of legally sufficient documentation inherent in the technology.

The following chart (Figure 2) gives an overview on how the three technological bases can be evaluated with regard to the above listed features.

Figure 2. Evaluation of the three technological bases

	Telephone	**Video-conferencing**	**Internet tools**
Synchronous communication possible	Y	Y	problematic
Asynchronous communication possible	N	Y	Y
Transmission of diagnostic material possible	N	Y	Y
Standardization	Y	Y	standardization not applicable for teleconsultation
Globally available	Y	N	potentially
Verification of partner's identity possible	N	Y	with use of special tools
Patient's rights and privacy preserved	Y	Y	with use of special tools
Inherent documentation	N	with minimal additional work	with minimal additional work

LEGAL AND SECURITY ASPECTS OF TELECONSULTATION

The introduction of current communication and information technologies in diagnostics and treatment does not change the legal basis of medicine, which has been established by the jurisdiction in several decades. However, the threats and risks change along with the use of medical telematics. In order to guarantee the observance of relevant medicolegal principles, increased technical and organizational measures must be taken [36]. Accuracy in previous planning and permanent control of organization and use are indispensable presuppositions for conducting teleconsultations in a legitimate way, the efficiency of a technical innovation being a product of organizational structures [37,38].

Since security technologies and legislation concerning telemedicine are evolving rapidly, the practice of teleconsultation has to be revised whenever necessary, so that compliance with the best possible standards can be achieved [39,40].

The Delineation of Responsibility between Primary Care Provider and Specialist

Authorization and competence: Health care professionals practising telemedicine must be authorized to practise medicine in the country or state in which they are located. They are responsible for the appropriate quality of their services (including equipment) [33].

The referring health care professional must choose a competent expert who may only accept giving advice in cases he is qualified in [41].

Principle of confidence versus assessment duties of the participants: According to the "principle of confidence", the consultant may rely upon the assumption that the health care professional in charge will provide all relevant findings accessible [41,42,43]. Nevertheless the consultant is obliged to evaluate carefully the transmitted material whether it is sufficient for decision finding [33]. If he recognizes obvious errors of his colleague who started the treatment, he is liable because of insufficient control of plausibility [32]. On the other hand, the referring health care professional may trust the expertise and experience of the consultant unless he makes a commonly obvious mistake of diagnosis [44].

Responsibility for treatment standards and methods: The standard of treatment has to be ensured regardless of the possibility of teleconsultation [32]. The health care professional leading the treatment remains responsible for his decisions and free to choose the method he prefers. He is not obliged to follow the advice of the consultant [32,33,41,42].

Liability: The referring health care professional is liable for damage whether he follows the consultants advice or not [42]. The consultant is involved in planning the therapeutic strategy and shares both medical and forensic responsibility according to the general liability principles [32,42,43].

Organizational responsibility: In case of errors which occur due to failures in communication or organization, principles of organizational responsibility apply primarily [32].

According to the health care professional's duty of professional carefulness, he is obliged to apply available technical and organizational security measures suitable for preventing unauthorized access to patient data during storage or transmission. The sender is liable for the integrity of the data as a reliable basis for medical decisions. The recipient has to identify the sender and has to check the integrity of the information transmitted [44,45].

It is strongly recommended that all institutions seeking or giving teleconsultation should establish an internal policy for teleconsultation in accordance with applicable laws. Conformity with or deviation from this policy must be recorded.

Documentation: Both sides are obliged to document the whole course of the teleconsultation properly and adequately (patient identification, questions of referring health care professional, quantity and quality of data transmitted, findings, recommendations or second opinion of the consultant) [32,33,42,43,44].

Data security and data protection: Unless special precautions are taken, illegal reading and manipulation of electronic data or falsifying the sender or recipient can be done easily and imperceptibly, creating problems of confidentiality and provability.

The necessity of data security calls for the use of best standard safety devices. Nevertheless encryption and digital signatures can not guarantee complete data protection, since future advances in cryptography might allow decoding of data that seem well protected today [32,46].

The following goals can be achieved by using public key infrastructure (PKI) for digital signatures, thus improving the development of reliable network security [37]:

1. Authenticity: Mutual correct and provable identification of communication partners.
2. Integrity: No uncontrollable manipulations of the documents content can have occurred on the way of transmission.
3. Non-Repudiation: The sending and receiving of a message is prooved and can not be denied afterwards.
4. Privacy: Only the legitimate recipient can read the document.

For the purpose of evidence, data should be signed with a verifiable date stamp, if possible [4,44,47].

Contracts for teleconsultation services: A contract regulating the interactions and obligations between the health care professionals/institutions involved in teleconsultation should cover the following issues:

Policy of teleconsultation: Both sides should be obliged to work in accordance with their policy for teleconsultation specifying details of preparation, conduction, and interaction [47].

Liability insurance: For both sides the proof of liability insurance coverage for referring/giving teleconsultation must be part of the contract [35,48].

Reimbursement: Reimbursement must be agreed upon [35] considering technological expenses (costs of communicational connections, initial outlay and operating of equipment), an administration and coordination fee, and remuneration for medical service.

Cross-border aspects: To avoid collisions of different national legal standards, the participants should agree on a choice of law and stipulate a place of jurisdiction [32,37,42,44,48].

The Delineation of Responsibility between Primary Care Provider and Specialist with regard to the Patient

Product liability: Being liable for the patient, the health care professional can obtain compensation from the producer of the equipment or the operator of the network who caused the damage [46].

Documentation – patients records: Upon request, up-to-date and complete medical records must be available at any time at least for the duration of the legal preservation period (in Germany 10 years) or the limitation period for any action for damages (in Germany 30 years). Since technological standards become obsolete rapidly, records can only be kept decipherable for such a long time by checking them regularly and transferring them onto a new system if necessary [32,35,42,45].

As records that can be falsified easily have low conclusiveness in liability trials and the burden of proof is on the health care professionals or hospitals side if records are inadequate or lost, high reliability and security of electronic records must be achieved [45].

Data protection and professional security: National legislation for data protection differs widely; in regard to teleconsultation it is recommended to establish high standards in any place [35,44,49].

Data protection acts are based on the patients right of informational self-determination: Storage, processing and transmission of patient data referable to an individual person is forbidden unless it is ordered by a legal regulation or permitted by an effective consent of the patient. Technical and organizational security measures should prevent misuse of the patient's data [44,49,50,51,52].

To achieve a maximum of security, the amount of data transferred should be reduced to the minimum sufficient for the telemedical application. If using anonymity or pseudonymity for transmitting data for medical purposes, the patient's consent is not generally necessary [32,39].

For anonymizing data appropriately it is not sufficient just to erase the patient's name, as other details may allow a conclusion to his identity [51].

If data transfer is urgently necessary to prevent severe injury to life or health of a patient who is not able to articulate his wishes e.g. because of unconsciousness, health care professionals may decide on the basis of the patient's presumable consent, carefully considering benefits and risks [52].

The patient's informed consent is only valid if the patient has been given all necessary information and explanations in a preliminary conversation which must not be replaced by simply handing out a form.

The consent form must be signed by the patient and documented at the referral site in the patient's record [32,39]. The consent and its purpose has to be communicated to the consultant and recorded with the data [52].

For being effective, the patient's consent must relate to a specific incident of transmitting his data and specify [36,51] which data may be transferred (extent):

1. the addressee (name and address of the recipient; for practical reasons the patient might agree that the teleconsultation request can be passed on to a substitute).
2. the purpose of the transmission.

Moreover, the patient must be informed about the following, if applicable [32,33,39,48,50]:

1. alternatives to the data transfer and possible consequences if the patient refuses to agree to teleconsultation.
2. typical risks like unauthorized access to the patient's data and their further uncontrollable transmission, mismatch of pictures or findings, interruption of the data transmission caused by technical reasons (broken hard- or software at the site of the referring health care professional or the consultant, problems during data transmission) or political incidents (satellite transmission cut off).
3. additional fees for teleconsultation the patient possibly must pay.
4. cross-border aspects.

The determination which national law has to be applied (differing liability standards) and whether the jurisdiction should be at the location of the consulted expert or at the site of the patient, must be documented in the consent form [39,53].

If the referring health care professional can not assure that the domestic data protection specifications are preserved abroad as well, the patient must explicitly consent [32,45].

STEPS OF IMPLEMENTATION

Summarising the issues in this paper, it can be concluded that teleconsultation is a viable way in health care to improve communication and structures as well as to spread competence. The underlying definition restricts teleconsultation to communication of two (or more) health care professionals with the subject of treatment planning of a patient's case. This implies that teleconsultation can take place only among professionals. In this context, it is mandatory that proper and efficient integration into everyday work processes is realized. In order to document this, institutions practising teleconsultation are strongly urged to issue a policy regarding the use of teleconsultation. On the other hand, such a policy is a means to be internally explicit about the applicable legal issues and identify cases in which contractual regulations beyond the ones outlined by the policy have to be found. The external contacts of an institution using teleconsultation ought to be formally agreed upon internally by means of the policy and externally by means of contracts. The patient's regards have to be respected and formally documented using a consent form. Thus, with the introduction of proper formal instruments, the introduction of technological innovation can give benefits to all involved groups and it can be done in a legally viable way.

The following steps outline a viable and safe way to introduce teleconsultation in an institution:

1. Decide, if teleconsultation should be performed, following a needs assessment and a sustainability committment.
2. Identify and regulate the legal and security issues applicable.
3. Decide on the technology to use and acquire it.
4. Develop and issue a policy, make contracts with partners for regular consultation.
5. Install and test the technology, implement the support structure.
6. Educate the potential users in the use and workflow of teleconsultation, integration into everyday work process and policy (including the decision on the necessity of personal or depersonalized data to be used and a schedule for quality assessment).
7. Initiate teleconsultation services (include a payment process or mechanism).
8. Provide and extend teleconsultation services (including support, ongoing education for the users, documentation and reimbursement).
9. Monitor possible changes of legal and security issues, eventually modify the policy and notify the users about the modifications.
10. Evaluate the teleconsultation services, analyse the medical outcome and the economic effects.
11. Eventually modify the teleconsultation services and the policy (if necessary), with constant feedback.

The following list provides the most common causes for problems in the use of teleconsultation:

1. Lack of communicational infrastructure.
2. Differences in measurements for diagnoses, in coding of diagnoses, and in categories used to describe a patient's case (medical standards) (Telemedicine Practice Guidelines).
3. Incompatible technological systems (interoperability).
4. Lack of education in the use of the systems.
5. Reimbursement issues and legal uncertaincy.

Teleconsultation may have a major impact on medical practice as such on a local as well as on a global level. Therefore it is important to teach, train and apply this technology properly and according to principles that can be derived from appropriate applications.

This guideline should ease the use of information technology in health care concerning the special sector of teleconsultation.

Members of the panel:

E. Andrew Balas (USA), Marcello Bracale (Italy), Christian Dierks (Germany), Charles R. Doarn (USA), Ian Mc Donald (Australia), André Lacroix (Canada), Louis Lareng (France), James McGee (UK), Ronald C. Merrell (USA), Michael Nerlich (Germany), Yoich Ogushi (Japan), Yoshikazu Okada (Japan), Oleg I. Orlov (Russia), Dittmar Padeken (Germany), Sandra Prerost (Australia), Jay H. Sanders (USA), Richard Wootton (UK).

References

[1]   Simpson J, Doze S, Urness D, Hailey D, Jacobs P. Evaluation of a routine telepsychiatry service. *Journal of Telemedicine and Telecare* 2001;7(2):90-8

[2]   Battmann A, Knitza R, Janzen S, *et al.* Telemedicine: application of telepathology-remote microscopy for intraoperative diagnoses on frozen sections. *Studies in Health Technology and Informatics* 2000;77:1127-30

[3]   Chan FY, Soong B, Lessing K, *et al.* Clinical value of real-time tertiary fetal ultrasound consultation by telemedicine: preliminary evaluation. *Telemedicine Journal* 2000 Summer;6(2):237-42

[4]   Stieglitz SP, Gnann W, Schächinger U, Maghsudi M, Nerlich M. Telekommunikation in der Unfallchirurgie. *Chirurg* 1998; 69(11):1123-8

[5]   Jolliffe VM, Harris DW, Whittaker SJ. Can we savely diagnose pigmented lesions from stored video images? A diagnostic comparison between clinical examination and stored video images of pigmented lesions removed for histology. *Clinical and Experimental Dermatology* 2001 Jan;26(1):84-7

[6]   Sawyer MA, Lim RB, Wong SY, Cirangle PT, Birkmire-Peters D. Telementored laparoscopic cholecystectomy: a pilot study. *Studies in Health Technology and Informatics* 2000;70:302-8

[7]   McCue MJ, Hampton CL, Malloy W, Fisk KJ, Dixon L, Neece A. Financial analysis of telecardiology used in a correctional setting. *Telemedicine Journal and E-Health* 2000 Winter;6(4):385-91

[8]   Loane MA, Bloomer SE, Corbett R, *et al.* A randomized controlled trial assessing the health economics of realtime teledermatology compared with conventional care: an urban versus rural perspective. *Journal of Telemedicine and Telecare* 2001;7(2):108-18

[9]   Lamminen H, Lamminen J, Ruohonen K, Uusitalo H. A cost study of teleconsultation for primary-care ophthalmology and dermatology. *Journal of Telemedicine and Telecare* 2001;7(3):167-73

[10]   Yoo SK, Kim SH, Kim NH, *et al.* Design of a PC-based multimedia telemedicine system for brain function teleconsultation. *International Journal of Medical Informatics* 2001 May;61(2-3):217-27

[11]   Sable C, Roca T, Gold J, Gutierrez A, Gulotta E, Culpepper W. Live transmission of neonatal echocardiograms from underserved areas: accuracy, patient care, and cost. *Telemedicine Journal* 1999 Winter;5(4):339-47

[12]   Johnston B, Wheeler L, Deuser J, Sousa KH. Outcomes of the Kaiser Permanente Tele-Home Health Research Project. *Archives of Family Medicine* 2000 Jan;9(1):40-5

[13]   Tachakra S, Hollingdale J, Uche CU. Evaluation of telemedical orthopaedic speciality support to a minor accident and treatment service. *Journal of Telemedicine and Telecare* 2001;7(1):27-31

[14]   Mair F, Whitten P. Systematic review of studies of patient satisfaction with telemedicine. *British Medical Journal* 2000 Jun;320(7248):1517-20

[15]   Oakley AM, Kerr P, Duffill M, *et al,* Patient cost-benefits of realtime teledermatology - a comparison of data from Northern Ireland and New Zealand. *Journal of Telemedicine and Telecare* 2000;6(2):97-101

[16]   Aarnio P, Rudenberg H, Ellonen M, Jaatinen P. User satisfaction with teleconsultations for surgery. *Journal of Telemedicine and Telecare* 2000;6(4):237-41

[17]   McConnell ME, Steed RD, Tichenor JM, Hannon DW. Interactive telecardiology for the evaluation of heart murmurs in children. *Telemedicine Journal* 1999 Summer;5(2):157-61

[18]   Aarnio P, Jaatinen P, Hakkari K, Halin N. A new method for surgical consultations with videoconference. *Annales Chirurgiae et Gynaecologiae Fenniae* 2000;89(4):336-40

[19]   Meck JM, Munshi G, Plempel J, Amato S, Macedonia C. Cytogenetic analysis using telemedicine consultation: an improved means of providing expert cross-coverage. *Genetics in Medicine* 1999 Nov-Dec;1(7):328-31

[20]   Szymas J, Papierz W, Danilewicz M. Real-time teleneuropathology for second opinion of neurooncological cases. *Folia Neuropathologica* 2000;38(1):43-6

[21]   Bergmo TS. A cost-minimization analysis of a routine teledermatology service in Norway. *Journal of Telemedicine and Telecare* 2000;6(5):273-7

[22] Smythe J, Yolton RL, Leroy A, *et al*. Use of teleoptometry to evaluate acceptability of a rigid gas-permeable contact lens. *Optometry* 2001 Jan;72(1):13-8

[23] Paiva T, Coelho H, Araujo MT et al. Neurological teleconsultation for general practitioners. *Journal of Telemedicine and Telecare* 2001;7(3):149-54

[24] Lambrecht CJ, Canham WD, Gattey PH, McKenzie GM. Telemedicine and orthopaedic care. A review of 2 years of experience. *Clinical Orthopaedics and Related Research* 1998 Mar;348:228-32

[25] Plinkert PK, Plinkert B, Zenner HP. Telemedicine in otorhinolaryngology. Basic principles and possible applications. *HNO* 2000 Sep;48(9):639-44

[26] Thorley PJ, Beacock DJ, Trickett CA, Sivananthan UM. 18FDG SPECT to assess myocardial viability: initial experience at a hospital remote from a cyclotron. *Nuclear Medicine Communications* 2000 Aug;21(8):715-8

[27] Biermann E, Dietrich W, Standl E. Telecare of diabetic patients with intensified insulin therapy. A randomized clinical trial. *Studies in Health Technology and Informatics* 2000,77:327-32

[28] Boulanger B, Kearney P, Ochoa J, Tsuei B, Sands F. Telemedicine: a solution to the followup of rural trauma patients? *Journal of the American College of Surgery* 2001;192:447-452

[29] Wirthlin DJ, Buradagunta S, Edwards RA, et al, Telemedicine in vascular surgery: feasibility of digital imaging for remote management of wounds. *Journal of Vascular Surgery* 1998 Jun;27(6):1089-99

[30] Nerlich M, Balas EA, Schall T, Stieglitz SP, Filzmaier R, Asbach P, Dierks C, Lacroix A, Watanabe M, Sanders JH, Doarn CR, Merrell RC. Teleconsultation practice guidelines: Report from G8 Global Health Applications Subproject 4. *Telemedical Journal and E-Health* 2002, 8(4):411-18

[31] http://www.iom.edu/. Last checked 11 December 2002

[32] http://www.db-law.de/html/body_dgmr-english.html. Last checked 11 December 2002

[33] http://www.utu.fi/research/mircit/ethics.html. Last checked 11 December 2002

[34] http://www.health.qld.gov.au/qtn/guidelines.htm. Last checked 11 December 2002

[35] http://www.meditac.org/MedITAC/documents/reports/annualreport2000.pdf. Last checked 11 December 2002

[36] Goetz C. Die Herausforderung „Telematik im Gesundheitswesen". *Bayererisches Ärzteblatt* 1999;10:23

[37] Lacroix A. International concerted action on collaboration in telemedicine: G8 sub-project 4. *Studies in Health Technology and Informatics* 1999;64:12-9

[38] Nerlich M. Medicolegal issues in telesurgery (lecture). G8 Global Healthcare Forum, London 1999

[39] Dierks C, Feussner H, Wienke A, eds. *Rechtsfragen der Telemedizin. MedR Schriftenreihe Medizinrecht*, Springer Verlag, Berlin-Heidelberg, 2000

[40] Rienhoff O. The SIREN Legal Workshops: List of urgent legal actions for telemedicine. In: Nerlich M, Kretschmer R, eds. *The Impact of Telemedicine on Health Care Management*. IOS Press Amsterdam 1999

[41] Ulsenheimer K. *Arztstrafrecht in der Praxis*. 2nd edn. Müller Verlag, Heidelberg 1998

[42] Feussner H, Etter M, Siewert JR. Telekonsultation. *Chirurg* 1998;Nov;69(11),1129-1133

[43] Etter M, Feussner H, Siewert JR. Guidelines for teleconsultation in surgery. The German experience. *Surgical Endoscopy* 1999 Dec;13(12):1254-5

[44] Ulsenheimer K, Heinemann N. Rechtliche Aspekte der Teleradiologie. *Radiologe* 1997:4,313-321

[45] http://www.iid.de/forschung/studien/telematik/. Last checked 11 December 2002

[46] http://www.teletrust.de. Last checked 11 December 2002

[47] http://telemedicine.partners.org:8080/demo3. Last checked 11 December 2002

[48] Schöne K. Wer haftet? Telemedizin – Haftungsrechtliche Risiken ohne Versicherungsschutz. *Management & Krankenhaus* 1999;9:15-16

[49] http://www.kvb.de/prax-edv/merkrahm.htm. Last checked 11 December 2002

[50] http://www.hcp-protokoll.de/arbeit/arbeit.htm. Last checked 11 December 2002

[51] Keller H. Ärztliche Schweigepflicht, Datenschutz in der Arztpraxis, Sicherheit der Praxis-EDV. *Broschüre der Kassenärztlichen Vereinigung Bayerns*, 2nd edn. Muenchen 1997

[52] Ulsenheimer K, Heinemann N. Rechtliche Aspekte der Telemedizin - Grenzen der Telemedizin? *MedR Schriftreihe Medizinrecht* 1999;5,197-203

[53] Hoppe JF. Telemedizin und internationale Arzthaftung. *MedR Schriftreihe Medizinrecht* 1998;10, 462-468

Address for correspondence

Patrick Asbach, MD
Department of Trauma Surgery
University of Regensburg
93042 Regensburg, Germany
phone: +49 941 944 6805
fax: +49 941 944 6806
e.mail: patrick.asbach@klinik.uni-regensburg.de

Medical Telematics in Disaster Response

THOMAS BENNER[1], ULRICH SCHAECHINGER[2], MICHAEL NERLICH[1,2]

[1]*International Center for Telemedicine Regensburg,*
Regensburg Emergency Services Center at the University,
Josef-Engert-Strasse 9, 93053 Regensburg, Germany
[2]*Department of Trauma Surgery, University of Regensburg,*
Franz-Josef-Strauss Allee 11, 93053 Regensburg, Germany

Abstract. Introduction: Every year many disasters cause thousands of injuries, deaths, refugees. Depending on the kind of disaster (train/plane accident, flood, earthquake) not only an acute emergency medicine treatment but also general and family medicine and hospital treatment have to be safeguarded over a longer time-period in the disaster area.

Problem: Regarding to a lot of organizations, institutions and disaster teams taking part in the disaster assistance is there any lack of work or data flow in the medical treatment?

Methods: From the ODRA flood 1997, the high speed train crash in ESCHEDE 1998, the DANUBE flood 1999 and the ELBE flood in 2002 experience reports were collected. They were analysed with emphasis on data and work flow in the medical treatment and its command system: Standardised command structure? Communication problems? Used communication lines? Language problems? Medical Intelligence distribution? Use of Patient Tracking System? Triage problems?

Results: The use of spoken radio communication causes transmission mistakes or misunderstandings and radio-overload and need connection-set-up-time for each call. Manual distribution of same data for many receivers using different communication lines causes a time shift in the up-to-date-information. Language problems during the ODRA flood between German and Polish people led to longer reaction times. Up-to-date triage results as well as up-to-date transportation and hospital information are necessary for medical evacuation. Compared with other reports about these disasters the quality of disaster management depends on the quality of communication and information.

Conclusion: The use of health telematics in disaster response helps to cope with the scenario. Modern technologies provide support for building up medical aid although the normal infrastructure is destroyed. To cope with disaster scenarios there are some telematic tools which can be used:
- Computer-based Command and Control System
- Telemedical support
- Data-ressources-network / Medical Intelligence
A further study is recommended to evaluate the real impact of using these telematic tools in a disaster.

Introduction

Every year many disasters cause thousands of injuries, deaths, refugees. In the year 1999 worldwide 14 big natural disasters with damage more than 1 Billion US Dollar were registered. Five of them caused more than one thousand deaths each.

The material and personal damage increases during the time: globally effective trends as urbanization, population growth, economic-technical progress and growing networks of the socio-technical systems lead to a worldwide increasing of damage.

In addition, the classically separation between natural disasters (earthquakes, volcanic eruption, floodings etc.) and human-made disasters (technical accidents, environment destruction etc.) more and more becomes very difficult [1].

The earthquakes in Turkey, the floodings in Venezuela and Mosambique as well as the floodings at Odra (1997) and Elbe (2002), the famine in Ethopia as well as the winter storms "Lothar" and "Martin" in Western Europe exemplary clarify the deficiencies of national and international disaster preparedness.

Such international as well as national disasters require premature and forecast plannings and remonstration. The most of the disasters simultaneously cause Mass Casualty Incidents (MCI). This means that the number of deaths and/or injuries overwhelm the normal community emergency response because there is always a strong disbalance between resource requirements and their availibility. So a not insignificant part present the planning and remonstration of the medical sector and health system [2].

Because Mass Casualty Incidents or disasters don't offer any pre-alarmtime or preparation time, detailed plannings for the mission are necessary in advance.

Accidents in the younger past as the high-speed train crash in ESCHEDE/Germany or the explosion of a factory for explosive devices in ENSCHEDE/Netherlands show ad-hoc appearing mass casualties with a lot of severe injured people, which have to receive a medical treatment in a very short time.

Accidents as the flooding of the river ODRA (1997) or ELBE (2002) show on the other hand long-term-disasters. Such long-term-disasters require a continous preparation of personal and material.

To coordinate all the different facilities and organizations involved in coping with the disaster there is an extensive demand of qualified Command, Control and Communication (C3).

In case of long-term-situations it is necessary to build up and maintain a medical treatment inside the destroyed areas, also considering the special hygienic and infectiological aspects.

Depending on the kind of disaster (train/plane accident, flood, earthquake) not only an acute emergency medicine treatment but also general and family medicine and hospital treatment have to be safeguarded over a longer time-period in the disaster area.

Problem

Because of many casualties in case of a disaster there is the basic rule, to do the best for the greatest number of victims at the right time and at the right place.

Often the final action has to be individually adapted to the not-present or destroyed infrastructure at the scene.

The disaster preparedness in Germany provides rescue means depending on the size of the Mass Casualty Incident in three categories. The Professional Emergency Medical Service (EMS) will be supported by Regional Medical Task Forces. Volunteer Disaster Teams then complete the system. All affected parties and their standby Mass-Casualty-Material and Vehicles are part of Disaster Management Plans which also include an established Structure for On-Site-Command and interdisciplinary training to verify periodic updates.

The structured order of the area contains a Triage Area and a separate Treatment Area near the scene. After the first treatment there will be transport to hospitals. This prevents from taking the disaster from the scene to the hospital (Figure 1).

Figure 1. Structured order of the area

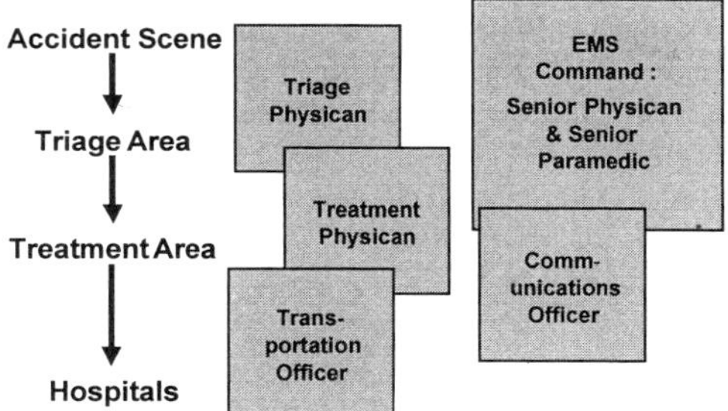

In case of a disaster the Command Post is the center of the different communication lines. Every sector on the scene, different dispatch or rescue coordination centers, hospitals, the government with its ressources, e.g. the Armed Forces, have to be connected in a functional system (Figure 2) [3].

Figure 2. Communication structure

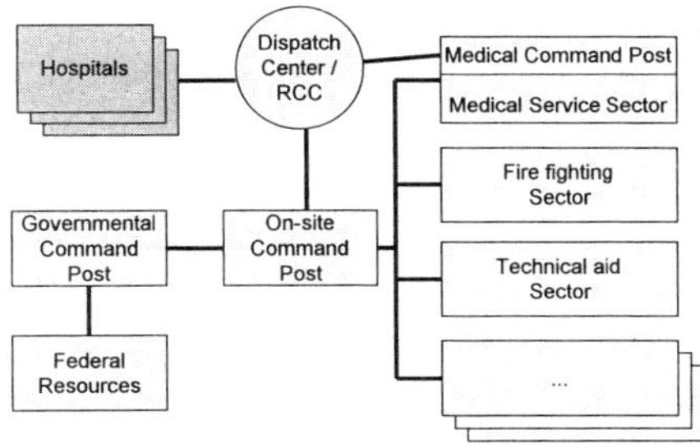

Regarding to a lot of organizations, institutions and disaster teams taking part in the disaster assistance and to the necessary coordination the question was raised if there is any lack of work or data flow in the medical treatment.

From the ODRA flood 1997, the high speed train crash in ESCHEDE 1998, the DANUBE flood 1999 and the ELBE flood 2002 experience reports were collected. They were analysed with emphasis on data and work flow in the medical treatment and its command system: Standardised command structure? Communication problems? Used communication lines? Language problems? Medical Intelligence distribution? Use of Patient Tracking System? Triage problems?

Results

In Germany a lot of different disasters occured in the past. The air show crash in Ramstein in the year 1988 brought up a lot to awareness and changed a lot in the response of a Mass Casualty Incident and its Command, Control and Communication structures in Germany.

During the past five years a lot of very big floodings (Odra 1997; Danube 1999; Elbe 2002) and the biggest crash in the history of the German railway show the two big differences of disasters.

The High-Speed-Train on its way from the southern to the northern part of Germany crashed into a bridge near the village of Eschede on the sunny morning of june 3rd, 1998. The train was 358 metres long and had 759 seats. The crash caused 96 dead and 108 injured casualties, mostly very badly injured. About 1800 (!) rescue and salvage workers and 39 rescue helicopters managed it to transport all the injured patients after three hours to 22 clinics in a range of maximum 150 kilometres [4].

Such ad-hoc disasters show that there is no time to prepare for this special incident. But on the other hand it is a local scene and support from the region around is possible so only emergency treatment is necessary on the scene.

In contrast to this floodings show other conditions. On a length of approximately 250 kilometres along the rivers there are thousands of people at risk, e.g. Danube '99: >100.000. A lot of these people have to be evacuated, e.g. Elbe 2002: >50.000. During the Elbe flooding in 2002 there was the biggest hospital evacuation of the past 50 years. Eight hospitals with 3000 patients including critical ill patients had to be evacuated. The patients were transported to hospitals all over Germany by land and air medical evacuation. This shows that the infrastructure of the incident area is lost. To cope with these cases approximately 30.000 rescue and salvage workers had to cope with these Long-term-disasters for approximately three weeks [5,6].

The destroyed infrastructure leads to the problem of no regional support. The consequence is that not only Emergency Medicine but also General/Family Medicine has to safeguard in the area.

The bigger the number of involved rescue teams or the bigger the geographical size of the accident, the more command, control and communication is required.

In the context of an oral communication there will be problems or mixup during the information flow and an always up-to-date documentation is required parallel. So the necessary data and work flow in the present is restricted by different reasons.

The use of spoken radio communication causes transmission mistakes or misunderstandings and radio-overload and need connection-set-up-time for each call. Manual distribution of same data for many receivers using different communication lines causes a time shift in the up-to-date-information. Language problems during the ODRA flood between German and Polish people led to longer reaction times [7]. Up-to-date triage results as well as up-to-date transportation and hospital information are necessary for medical evacuation.

The coordinated treatment requires a lot of data. The collection of these informations will be difficult because of different documentation systems in use depending on the regional area. The data collection contains of Patient Identification (e.g. ID-No., Name), Triage category, Clinical Signs, Monitoring data, Medical Treatment and relevant Tactical Informations.

All the affected parties (Figure 3) need all or parts of the collected informations. So it is often the similiar data but for different use:

• Dispatch Center / Rescue Coordination Center (RCC)
    ⌈ Responsible for all involved vehicles (air, land, water)
    ⌈ Coordinating Hospital Capacities
• Hospitals
    ⌈ Preparing the Emergency Room
    ⌈ Providing Capacitiy for Medical Treatment, e.g. Surgical Procedures,
      ICU,Toxicology

• Family Assistance Centers
• Police / Public Affairs Services / Government
• Quality Management / Feedback
• Insurance Agencies

The present used methods cause the following problems in work flow [7]. Each of the problems can be solved by using modern technologies.

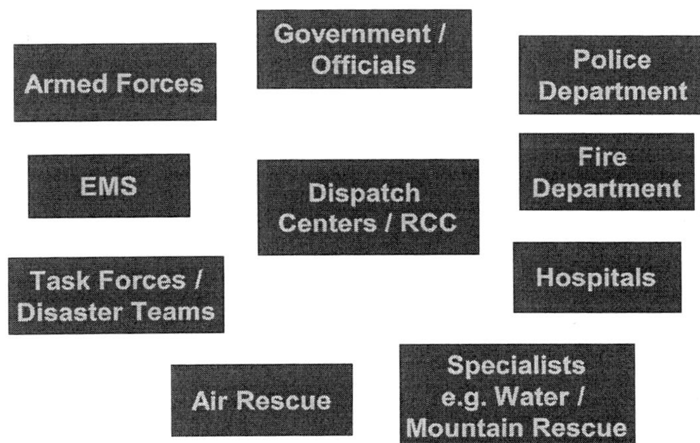

Figure 3. Affected parties.

1. The loss of information because of verbal communication via many instances can be solved by written data with digital adressing (like "e-mail").
2. Every call needs Connection-Set-Up-Time. With the "Fire and Forget"-method the user only puts the information into the electronic device and gives it the instruction to send and receive.
3. Use of digital Packet-data can avoid Radio-Overload.
4. Mobility combined with the necessary bandwith, e.g. to set up an on-site-command can be achieved by using satellite communication (SatCom), Wireless Network (WLAN) or digital radio standards as TETRA.
5. Automatic Data-Exchange leads to realtime information-updates.
6. Computerized translation modules can improve the understanding in spite of different languages, e.g. refugee camps.
7. The use of international standards lets systems of different organizations work together.
8. Tele-Access to databases provides the best knowledge of all required data for all affected parties and makes Medical Intelligence possible.

Conclusion

With the use of health telematic applications there is the possibility by the use of cable or wireless communication-lines to provide necessary informations independent of time and area.

To optimize the treatment this is additionally very valuable to provide knowledge of the different special fields of medicine.

The use of health telematics in disaster response helps to cope with the scenario [8]. Modern technologies provide support for building up medical aid although the normal infrastructure is destroyed.

To connect the levels of user and expert the needs can be summarized to "Three Pillars for Telematical Support in Disaster Response" (Figure 4).

Figure 4. Three Pillars for Telematical Support in Disaster Response

Specialist / Clinic	Command Post	Officials / Institutes
Med. Diagnosis Monitoring Therapy **„Telemedicine"** Teleconsultation, Telearchiving	Medical Command **Safeguarding the Commanding ability** -Patient-Tracking -Command -Control -Communication	**Medical Intelligence / Databases** -Epidemiology -data/fact sheets -Algorithms / SOP

Rescue Teams   EMS Command   Emergency Physicans

Treatment Areas   „MedicPoints"

The core of a sufficient disaster response is the Command, Control and Communication. A lot of informations collected during a disaster have to be distributed to a lot of receivers even in different languages. To solve the data flow it is possible using health telematics for patient tracking and -movement. For a better work flow the status of the Emergency Medical Service (EMS) and hospitals and situation reports will be presented digital. The high organizational expenditure can be reduced by the connection of data processing and telecommunication (= telematics). This will reduce report lines and avoid repetitions of oral dictations or paper copies of informations. For the following work steps standardized digital reports can be used: demand for further teams, material or vehicles; situation reports of the involved teams; assignment of the areas of responsibility; coordination of the transport; triage documentation of the senior physician; patient tracking and movement; survey of all hospitals [9].

For the realization of these steps small computers, notepads or notebooks are necessary. They have to communicate by wireless technics with each other and with a server. Wireless connections depend on the available infrastructure. The biggest independence will be reached by the use of own systems, for example a Wireless-Local-Area-Network (WLAN).

The computer can furthermore use a barcode-reader to improve the patient tracking and a card-reader to use the digital information on the patient's insurance card. In combination with satellite navigation (GPS) injured people or incident sites can be reached by coordinates. A digital camera can send live pictures from the scene to evaluate and to document the situation. The Medical Assistance Teams on the scene can use such portable devices as their "electronic life belt" [10,11]

Telemedical issues transfer standardised medical data so that tele-consultation, tele-archiving, tele-assistance is possible. The central problem is that the destroyed infrastructure includes clinics and practices. Because during triage more patients are rated more critical as they really are, repetition of triage is recommended during the treatment. Therefore it could be useful to triage victims for medical evacuation or to monitor patients on the local scene without bringing them to special medical facilities. On the increasing danger of infectious diseases additional attention has to be payed. According to this telemedical support for vaccination tasks is possible. (During a flooding more than 10.000 volunteers got vaccinations in the first week.) The physicians working on the scene will come from different medical specialties. With the possibility of presenting the patient to other experts via teleconsultation many different special fields can take part in diagnosis and send recommendations for treatment. This leads to an easier decision finding.

With a mobile or portable Videoteleconferencing-System and the possibility to transmit ECG, Ultrasound and other sources it is possible for the medical crew at a "MedicPoint" to get support by experts of all medical fields. Furthermore the data can collected and archived by a server placed out of the destroyed area (Tele-Archiving) [12,13,14].

Health telematics include the presentation of up-to-date data of nuclear, biological or chemical warfare, epidemiology, standard-operating-procedures (SOP), alghorithms and all other informations which are useful for the treatment of patients at any place on the scene. This network of knowledge improves the Medical Intelligence which is important for an adaption to all circumstances and influences to the incident [15,16].

To use the advantages of health telematics a network of desktop computers, laptops, notepads, personal digital assistants (PDA) is required. They have to be linked by using a redundant server system to provide a work flow without loss of data (Figure 5).

Figure 5. Future Work Flow Vision

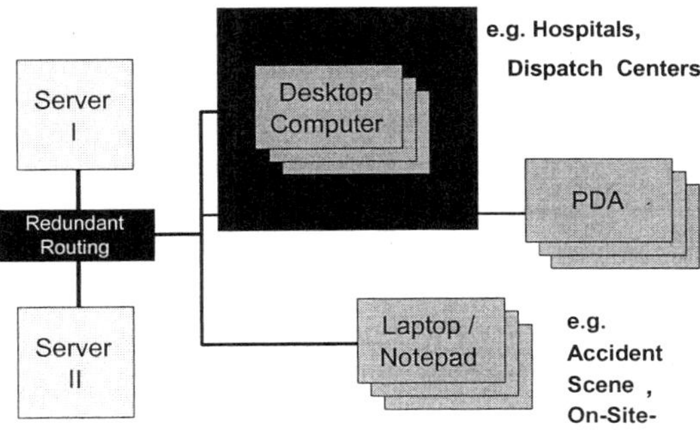

Because of the independence of time and geographical location health telematics can support in Hazardous Material-Casualties. The central problem in these incidents is the strict separation between contaminated and non-contaminated area. Telematics can provide:

• Teleconference to improve communication between inside and outside the contaminated area
• Tele-Consultation to assist specialists/Fact Finding Teams inside the contaminated area
• transmitting pictures to outside for evaluation and documentation
• Database-Access: e.g. Hazardous-/ nuclear-, biological-, chemical-(NBC-)Material / Antidotas
• transmitting measurement results

These results present the theoretical evaluation of the use of health telematics in disaster response. Now a further study is recommended to evaluate the real impact of using telematic tools in a disaster.

References

[1]   German Committee for Disaster Reduction within the International Strategy for Disaster Reduction (ISDR): Annual Report 1999.
[2]   Bundesministerium des Innern: Katastrophenmedizin. Leitfaden für die ärztliche Versorgung im Katastrophenfall. Berlin 2001.
[3]   Crespin UB, Neff G: Handbuch der Sichtung. Stumpf und Kossendey. Edewecht 2000.
[4]   Oestern HJ et al.: Facts about the Disaster at Eschede. J Orthop Trauma, 2000 14(4)
[5]   Löffler D.: Hochwasserkatastrophe in Bayern 1999. Probleme der Führung bei Großschadensereignissen und Katastrophen. Notfallvorsorge 2000 (4)
[6]   Jahrhundertflut in Deutschland: eine Chronologie. Feuerwehrfachzeitschrift 2002 (10): 577-603
[7]   Ministerium des Innern des Landes Brandenburg, Referat Brand- und Katastrophenschutz: Hochwasserkatastrophe Juli/August 1997 an der Oder. Erfahrungsbericht. Potsdam 1997.
[8]   Jäckel A: Telemedizinführer Deutschland. Ausgabe 2000. Deutsches Medizin Forum, Bad Nauheim 1999
[9]   Plischke M et al.: Telemedical Support of Prehospital Emergency Care in Mass Casualty Incidents. Eur J Med Res 1999 (4): 394-398
[10] Schaechinger U et al.: Notfall-Organisations- und Arbeitshilfe (NOAH): Informationsmanagement in der präklinischen Notfallmedizin. Notfall 2001 27(3)
[11] Schaechinger U et al.: NOAH--A mobile emergency care system. Eur J Med Res 2000 (1):13-8
[12] Wickenhöfer R et al.: Telemedizin in der Bundeswehr. Wehrmedizin und Wehrpharmazie 2001 (2)
[13] Bolte M, Wilke D: Grundlagen der Telemedizin. Wehrmedizin und Wehrpharmazie 2001 (3)
[14] Anzinger G et al.: Einsatz der Telemedizin bei Auslandeinsätzen - Vorstellung von zwei Fallbeispielen. Wehrmed Mschr 2000 4(2-3)
[15] East Carolina University, Center for Health Sciences Communication: Evaluation of Telemedicine used in a simulated Disaster Response. United States Navy Strong Angel Exercise. http://www.telemed.med.ecu.edu/2001/strong/
[16] Balch DC, West VL: Telemedicine used in a simulated disaster response. Stud Health Technol Inform 2001 (81): 41-5

Address for correspondence

Thomas Benner
International Center for Telemedicine (ICT) Regensburg
Regensburg Emergency Services Center at the University
Telemedizinisches Service Zentrum (TMSZ)
Josef-Engert-Strasse 9
93053 Regensburg, Germany
phone: +49 941 943 1784
fax: +49 941 943 1853
e.mail: thomas.benner@stud.uni-regensburg.de

Architecture and Tools for Open, Interoperable and Portable EHRs

BERND BLOBEL

Institute of Biometrics and Medical Informatics, Otto-von-Guericke University Magdeburg,
Leipziger Strasse 44, 39120 Magdeburg, Germany

Abstract. Electronic Health Record (EHR) systems provide the kernel application of health information systems and health networks which should be independent of complexity, localisation constraints, platforms, protocols, etc. Based on shared care information systems' requirements for high level interoperability, a generic component architecture has been introduced. For implementing, running and maintaining acceptable and useable health information systems components, all views of the ISO Reference Model – Open Distributed Processing have to be considered. Following the Model Driven Architecture paradigm, a reference model as well as concept-representing domain models both independent of platforms must be specified, which are combined and harmonised as well as automatically transferred into platform-specific models using appropriate tools.

Introduction

Health information systems supporting shared care with its characteristics of distribution, communication, and co-operation have to be highly interoperable independent of complexity, localisation constraints, platforms, etc. Therefore, such systems have to meet systems' requirements of openness, scalability, portability, distribution on the Internet level and must be generally based on international standards. Furthermore, shared care information systems have to provide appropriate security and privacy services. Regarding such systems' communication and co-operation, different levels of interoperability can be distinguished. Those interoperability levels are ranging from simple data exchange, meaningful data exchange with agreed vocabulary, functional interoperability with agreed communicating applications' behaviour, or finally service-oriented interoperability directly invoking the applications' services. For more details see [1].

Electronic Healthcare Record Systems

In healthcare, information that is valid has to be dealt with, and must therefore be available for, the patient's entire life-time. In that context, the extension of the domain as well as the speed of change in concepts and practice is an important impediment. The health system has a special need for communicating and also using health information concerning patients' care data for statistical purposes such as cost trends, epidemiology, demography and public health, as well as for education and research. As an adequate means for recording, storing, processing and communicating patient-related medical information, the electronic healthcare record has been defined, specified and standardised (e.g. [2]).

Following the definitions of Thomas Beale [3], an EHCR is a repository of information about a patient's health that is stored in a computer-readable format. The EHCR results from care processes and controls care processes, for example, it derives alerts, supports decision-making, etc. An EHCR system is a set of components that provide the mechanisms for creating, using, storing and retrieving a patient record. The EHCR architecture itself is a model of generic properties that are required for any electronic medical record to make this record a communicable, complete, useful, effective and ethically and legally binding record, which maintains its integrity over time, independent of platforms and systems, as well as national peculiarities. EHCRs have to be unambiguous, complete, context-preserving, extendable and multilingual, etc. Internationally, three standard concepts have been established for EHCR specifications and implementations: the component-oriented single model approach [2], the component-oriented dual model approach [4,5,6] and component-oriented services [1,7]. The first two approaches pursue a data integration, embed concepts into structures – in the case of the single model approach – or specify and implement them using archetypes – in the case of the dual model approach – as well as make functionalities such as workflow concepts, and alert mechanisms that are derived from the available data. The third approach realises functional integration, i.e. interoperability, due to the architecture paradigm that is deployed [1].

EHR architectures and systems cannot be introduced in one step. Starting in the sixties, the definition and establishment of EHR is a long-lasting challenge. Figure 1 shows the model for developing the EHCR as a kernel application in hospitals or in shared care systems, respectively [8]. This will happen in a stepwise procedure. The first three steps concern the hospital internal view, the fourth step enables communication and co-operation between healthcare establishments (HCEs), and the fifth opens the view of a personal life record including preventive aspects and social affairs, etc.

Figure 1. Model of EHCR Development

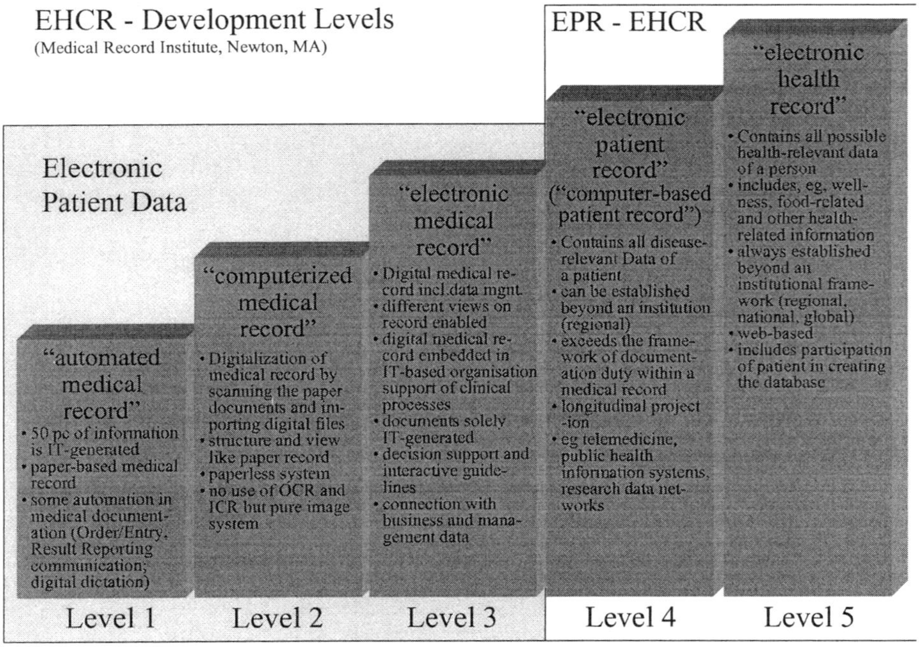

If traditional administrative solutions are based on the processing of data with restricted automated interpretation and build at a rather static context, medical department systems and also advanced management systems require an orientation on information, as well as their flexible, context-related processing and provision. Based on the data in common – comprehensive EHCR, repository and data warehouse – it is the task of departmental systems to put the corresponding concepts, contexts and functionalities on the data. In order to ensure its quality and integrity, the information should be recorded and managed at the place of origin. Redundancies should be avoided. Therefore, EHCRs are virtual solutions that are centralised logically but not physically. Both evolutions – of integration and kernel applications – are essential for developing information and communication technology (ICT) strategies in healthcare.

A Future Proof EHR Architecture

During the last five to ten years, different advanced EHR architectures have been developed which have been summarised, e.g., in [1,9]. Following, an advanced future proof architectural approach to health information systems including EHR systems will be presented which has harmonised and improved the currently available solutions.

Component Based Architectures

Information systems intend to reflect legal, organisational, functional, technological, and content constraints. Furthermore, they have to enable interoperability not only at data but also at functional or even knowledge level. The architecture meeting these challenges should consist of generic, encapsulated, persistent pieces which are accessible via interfaces and inherit or override their properties. These properties are met by objects. While objects are defined originally as

$$\text{Object} = \text{attributes} + \text{operations} \tag{1}$$

the constraints are represented by object-object interactions and cannot be invoked via interfaces. Components on the other hand are characterised by

$$\text{Component} = \text{attributes} + \text{operations} + \text{structural constraints} + \text{operational} \tag{2}$$
$$\text{constraints} + \text{events} + \text{multi-interfaces} * \text{scenarios} + \text{safety} +$$
$$\text{reliability} + \text{security} + ...$$

Therefore, the EHR architecture has to meet the component paradigm.

The different EHCR approaches established have been harmonised combining modern development paradigms and the huge domain knowledge expressed in other models, standards and R&D-project outcome. This has been done using the generic component approach developed by the Magdeburg Medical Informatics Department at mid-nineties [10]. Starting point of the approach is the ISO Reference Model – Open Distributed Processing (ISO RM-ODP) [11].

The ISO Reference Model – Open Distributed Processing

Depending on the requirements and needs of the user and his underlying models, concepts, etc., information systems have to offer different views on the real world within their development, implementation, and maintenance phase. For keeping the systems manageable in the phases mentioned, different level of granularity of considering the real world systems can be considered. In order to meet all of the possible requirements, an information system will enable all of the necessary views (different levels of abstraction) on the system that is supported, at all levels of granularity that are required. According to the ISO RM-ODP, the views concern the enterprise view, the information view, the computational view, the engineering view and the technology view. The granularity concerns concepts, relations network, aggregations and details. Regarding the corporate structure, the whole healthcare establishment, the relation between structural units, the departments, and procedural steps can be distinguished.

Model Driven Architectures

Regarding concepts, advanced architectural approaches group systems and their components into domains with the same objective of keeping development and maintenance of complex health information systems manageable. A domain is characterised by components of a system grouped by common legal, organisational, logical, and technical properties. This could be done for common policies (policy domains) which are discussed in section 3, for common environments (environment domains), or common technology (technology domains) [12]. To enable context-sensitive information system architectures as well as the presentation of domain-specific or view-specific knowledge, components and their corresponding object adapter must be managed in a flexible way according to the users' needs. The emerging CORBA 3 environment provides specifications and methods to fulfil those requirements [13]. Using these methods such as valuetypes, persistent state services, portable object adapter, or CORBA component model, the models describing the different levels of abstraction and granularity mentioned above can be developed and implemented. Starting from platform independent models and platform independent domain models dealing with the domain specific knowledge expressed as constraints and relations, platform specific models as well as platform specific domain models are derived from the unspecific ones. The unspecific models are called object models. Specific models have to meet constraints. Models representing constraints in content, datatypes, procedures, etc., are called archetypes. Therefore, specific models are called archetype models. Object model and archetype models can be derived from complex models or vice versa. Instantiation of archetype models and object model are bound together at runtime. The archetypes concern any concepts such as medical specialities, organisational restrictions or personal peculiarities. Thus, different concepts within one view (abstraction level) or related to different view on a system can be specified. For binding the models in an unambiguous way, digital signature mechanisms might be deployed. This way for providing safety of the EHCR components will be extended towards reliability and security services. In that context, concepts for establishing both communication and application security services must be specified in archetypes. In actual EHR approaches, the Unified Modeling Language (UML) is used to model the components and the Extensible Markup Language (XML) schemata are deployed to express the different views explained before.

Components can perform state transitions regarding their level of granularity or their level of abstraction, respectively. The state transition has to follow strict rules for preserving consistency and integrity of the system and its views [3]. This state transition is realised through specialisation, generalisation, or association as well as by different constraints dedicated to the component. Composition or decomposition might be provided by separating at least some constraints from the basic component (Figure 2).

Figure 2. State Transitions within the Abstraction-Granularity Matrix of Component Systems

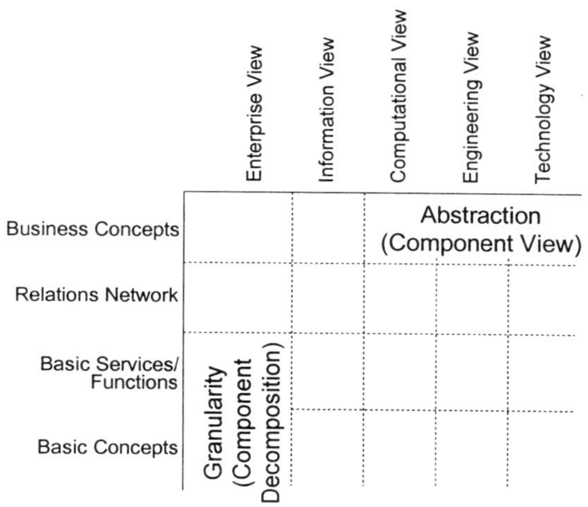

The HARP[1] EHR Implementation

According to the generic component model [1,10], all views, information content, functionality, implementation environment, and underlying technology but also the proper level of granularity might be modelled in a consistent way. In this way services and the complexity of the running application component can be defined according to the application environment and the user needs. Services concern entry, processing, and presentation of data but also the enforcement of underlying policy for communication and co-operation. The generic component model enables claims change management (viewpoint of the system) and the resolution of the component's complexity by the transition to less complex sub-components as shown in figure 2. Each specific model in the abstraction-granularity space reflects one specific archetype. A theoretical consideration on consistency for state transitions within the generic model has been provided in [1,10].

The description of the components according to equation (2) is established in archetype schemas using the XML (Extensible Markup Language) standard set. Related to granularity and technology viewpoint, mobile computing has to meet special requirements which are easily enabled by this dynamic selective approach of the proper state of a complex system.

Within the HARP project [14], partners from Greece, Germany, Norway, United Kingdom, and the Netherlands specified, developed and implemented the HARP Cross Security Platform (HCSP) for Internet based secure component systems as well as the development methodology and the development tools needed have been specified.

---

[1] The HARP (Harmonisation for the Security of Web Technologies and Applications) project (Project Number: IST-1999-10923) was funded by the European Commission within the Information Society Technologies (IST) Programme Framework

Security Services in the OpenEHR Context

As already mentioned, the archetypes describe conceptual, contextual, organisational, functional, but also legal and ethical framework of the EHCR system and its behaviour. Such framework is also called policy. Archetypes define the domain-specific constraints to be established. Therefore, archetypes enable the description of policies. By refining archetypes, detailed specifications for security services such as authorisation and access control management can be specified and at runtime instantiated. Following the GEHR/ openEHR approach [4,5], the overall policy as well as its refinements in special policies and detailed security services sense should be specified in archetype models and expressed in XML schema [15]. The generic meta-models have to be specified using the XML Schema standard.

The HARP Cross Security Platform

The HARP project's objective is building up entirely secure applications in client-server environments over the Web. Real interoperability leads to a closer connection of both communication and application security services. Communication security services comprise strong mutual authentication and accountability of principals involved, integrity, confidentiality and availability of communicated information as well as some notary's services. As a result of the authentication procedure, authorisation for having access to the other principal has to be decided. Application security services concern accountability, authorisation and access control regarding data and functions, integrity, availability, confidentiality of information recorded, processed and stored as well as some notary's services and audit.

To provide platform independence of solutions in HARP as a real three tiers architecture, the design pattern approach of developing a middleware-like common cross platform (HCSP) has been used. In HCSP, platform-specific security features have been isolated. Using an abstraction layer, communication in different environment is enabled. According to the component paradigm, an interface definition of a component providing a platform-specific service specifies how a client accesses a service without regard of how that service is implemented. So, the HCSP design isolates and encapsulates the implementation of platform-specific services behind a platform-neutral interface as well as reduces the visible complexity. Only a small portion has to be rewritten for each platform The solutions concern secure authentication as well as authorisation of principals even not registered before, deploying proper Enhanced Trusted Third Party (ETTP) services [1]. Especially, it helps to endorse policies by mapping them on processing components. For that reason, HARP components follow the specification of equation (2).

HARP's generic approach implements several basic principles. HARP's solution of embedding security into any application to be instantiated over the web-based environment outlined above is based on object oriented programming principles. It is based on Internet technology and protocols solely. The trustworthiness needed has been provided by applying only certified components which are tailored according to the principal's role. In fine-grained steps, it establishes its complete environment required, avoiding any external services possibly compromised. After strong mutual authentication based on smartcards and TTP services [16,17], the security infrastructure components are downloaded and installed to be used for implementing the components needed to run the application as well as to transfer data input and output. The SSL (Secure Socket Layer) protocol deployed to initiate secure sessions is provided by the Java Secure Socket Extension API. The applets and servlets for establishing the local client and the open remote database access facilities communicate using the XML standard set including XML Digital Signature. Because messages and not single items are signed, the messages are archived separately for accountability reasons meeting the legislation and regulations for health.

Policies are dynamically interpreted and adhered to the components. All components applied at both server and client site are checked twice against the user's role and the appropriate policy: first in context of their selection and provision and second in context of their use and functionality.

Applet security from the execution point of view is provided through the secure downloading of policy files, which determine all access rights in the client terminal. This has to be seen on top of the very desirable feature that the local, powerful, and versatile code is strictly transient and subject to predefined and securely controlled download procedures. All rights corresponding to predefined roles are subject to personal card identification with remote mapping of identity to roles and thereby to corresponding security policies with specific access rights.

For realising the services and procedures described, an applet consists of the sub-components GUI and interface controller, smartcard controller, XML signing and XML processing components, communication component applying the Java SSL extension, and last but not least the data processing and activity controller. Beside equivalent sub-components and an attribute certificate repository at the server side, policy repository, policy solver and authorisation manager have been specified and implemented as a "light weight" Resource Access Decision service (CORBA: RAD) [17].

After exchanging certificates and establishing the authenticated secure session, servlet security is provided from the execution point of view through listing, selecting and finally executing the components to serve the user properly. By establishing an authenticated session that persists for all service selections, a single-sign-on approach can be realised.

HARP enables the implementation of openEHR [5] in a convincing way. Using the open environment of certified Java™ components, portability of the HARP solution to any platform is guaranteed. In the server-centric approach, a web-accessible middleware has been chosen based on its support of basic security functionality, e.g., MICO/SSL., Apache Web server with mod_ssl, Apache JServ, and Apache Jakata Tomcat. Combining the server-centric approach of HCSP, its server-centric approach and the network-centric VPN behaviour, the completely distributed HARP Cross Security Platform has been designed.

Harmonising the HARP Approach and OpenEHR

The HARP approach enables the implementation of any EHR component following constraints defined in archetype models and expressed in XML schema. The HCSP facilitate the instantiation of those components by combining both specifications in the sense of certified components. So, any granularity, any constraint in the sense of domain knowledge, organisational structure, underlying policy, technological requirements for structure and presentation providing portability, etc. is supported properly.

The development of HARP rules underlying the XML messages which establish the HARP components (servlets and applets) is based on UML models. Within the HARP project developed independently from openEHR, these models reflect archetypes. For enhancing the current openEHR specification by security archetypes, a harmonisation in concepts and especially terminology used must be performed.

Conclusions

EHR architecture and subsequently specified and implemented EHR systems have to meet the shared care paradigm establishing openness, interoperability, scalability, and portability for providing any needed and permitted information to any authorised user at time, location, and format required, including mobile devices. Furthermore, EHR systems have to comply with comprehensive security solutions solely based on available and emerging standards. Actual EHR architecture standards comparably presented in the paper move in the direction requested. Emerging common projects harmonise the different approaches towards a "global" openEHR.

The European HARP project specified and implemented open portable EHR systems enriched with enhanced TTP services and comprehensive development strategies for establishing fine grained application security services. Constraints specified can be bound to components at runtime, enabling different views or supporting specific domain knowledge concepts. By binding attribute certificates to components appropriate policies can be enforced. These constraints such as, e.g., certificates are interpreted at both server and client sides using authorisation services. The HARP Cross Security Platform is solely based on standards including the XML standard set for the establishment of EHR clients and servers as well as their communication.

Acknowledgement

The author is in debt to the European Commission for funding and to the EHR community as well as to the HARP project partners for their support and their kind co-operation.

References

[1]   Blobel B. Analysis, Design and Implementation of Secure and Interoperable Distributed Health Information Systems. Series Studies in Health Technology and Informatics, Vol. 89. IOS Press, Amsterdam, 2002.
[2]   CEN ENV 13606 "Health Informatics – Electronic Healthcare Record Communication", 1999
[3]   Beale T. An Interoperable Knowledge Methodology for Future-Proof Information Systems, 2001
[4]   GEHR Project: www.gehr.org
[5]   openEHR Consortium. www.openehr.org
[6]   CEN ENV 13606 "Health Informatics – Electronic Health Record Communication", Revision
[7]   Blobel B. Concepts and Solutions for Future-Proof Health Information Systems and Health Networks. In: Blobel B, Pharow P (Edrs.) Advanced Health Telematics and Telemedicine. The Magdeburg Expert Summit Textbook. Series Studies in Health Technology and Informatics, Vol. 96. IOS Press, Amsterdam (2003).
[8]   Medical Record Institut: www.medrecinst.com
[9]   Blobel B. Comparing Concepts for Electronic Healthcare Record Architectures. In: Surján G, Engelbrecht R, McNair P (Edrs.) Health Data in the Information Society, pp 118-122. Series Studies in Health Technology and Informatics, Vol. 90. IOS Press, Amsterdam (2002).
[10] Blobel B. Application of the Component Paradigm for Analysis and Design of Advanced Health System Architectures. *International Journal of Medical Informatics* **60** (3) (2000) 281-301.
[11] ISO/IEC 10746-2 "Information Technology – Open Distributed Processing – Reference Model: Part 2: Foundations".
[12] Object Management Group, Inc.: The CORBA Security Specification. Framingham: Object Management Group, Inc., 1995, 1997.
[13] Siegel J. Quick CORBA3. Wiley Computer Publishing, John Wiley & Sons, Inc., New York, Chichester, Weinheim, Brisbane, Singapore, Toronto, 2001.
[14] The HARP Consortium: http://www.ist-harp.org

[15] Blobel B, Nordberg R. Privilege Management and Access Control in Shared Care IS and EHR. In: Baud R, Fieschi M, LeBeux P, Ruch P (Edrs.) The New Navigators: From Professionals to Patients, pp 251-256. Series Studies in Health Technology and Informatics, Vol. 95. IOS Press, Amsterdam (2003).
[16] Blobel B, Pharow P. Security Infrastructure of an Oncological Network Using Health Professional Cards. In: van den Broek L, Sikkel AJ (Edrs.) Health Cards '97, pp 323-334. Series in Health Technology and Informatics Vol. 49. IOS Press, Amsterdam (1997).
[17] ISO DTS 17090 "Public Key Infrastructure, Part 1 – 3", 2001.

Address for correspondence

PD Dr. Bernd Blobel
Institute of Biometrics and Medical Informatics
Otto-von-Guericke University Magdeburg
Leipziger Strasse 44
39120 Magdeburg, Germany
phone: +49 391 6713542
fax: +49 391 6713536
e.mail: bernd.blobel@mrz.uni-magdeburg.de

Telemedicine in Extreme Environments: Analogs for Space Flight

CHARLES R. DOARN

*Executive Director, Medical Informatics and Technology Applications Consortium
Assistant Professor. Department of Surgery, Virginia Commonwealth University,
PO Box 980480, Richmond, VA 23298-0480, USA*

Abstract. The integration of telecommunications and information systems into health care delivery in human space flight operations is not new. It has been an integral tool for over 45 years. During these past decades, numerous efforts have been conducted to further develop and promulgate telemedicine. The National Aeronautics and Space Administration (NASA) established a commercial space center in 1997, known as the Medical Informatics and Technology Applications Consortium (MITAC). MITAC has developed and conducted a variety of test beds in several international settings, including Russia, Ecuador and other extreme and remote environments. These test beds have been designed to evaluate and validate technologies and techniques that have application in the delivery and support of health care in unique environments. The characteristics of these test beds are analogous to what might be observed or experienced in low earth orbit or on space-based platform. These include intermittent communications, low bandwidth, level of competency of the front line health worker, etc. These test beds have led to new approaches for the delivery of health care as well as enhanced education. These experiences have been beneficial in the promulgation of telemedicine as an effective tool and have provided new ideals for space exploration as well terrestrial medicine. This paper will highlight MITAC's test beds and their relationship to space exploration.

Introduction

In 1969, when U.S. astronaut Neil Armstrong stepped on the moon, physicians in Houston, TX monitored his health status using telemedicine. In 1957, the Soviet Union launched that second man-made satellite, Sputnik 2. This satellite contained a dog, named Laika, as illustrated in Figure 1. Laika was monitored during the entire flight for physiological status [1]. Sending animals or even humans into the extreme environments of space was a tremendous challenge. There were many unknowns. Of course earlier explorers who were preparing to traverse vast oceans had no idea what challenges lay before them.

The Wright Brothers mastered flight 100 years ago. Humankind mastered the rocket and successfully landed men on the moon. The U.S. Space Shuttle with well over 1,000,000 parts operates in a highly efficient and integrated fashion. These complex problems do not always require complex solutions. Telemedicine solutions do not have to be complicated.

Using telemedicine as a tool in extreme environments requires an understanding of what such an environment is like. There are many places on earth that are similar to what space is like in terms of extremeness and remoteness. These environments are considered analogs for space flight [2,3]. Environments that are characterized as extreme, remote or isolated, can be in the developed and developing world, in the Antarctic, Mt. Everest, or your own home in large metropolitan area.

Figure 1. Laika encapsulated in the life support system for Sputnik 2

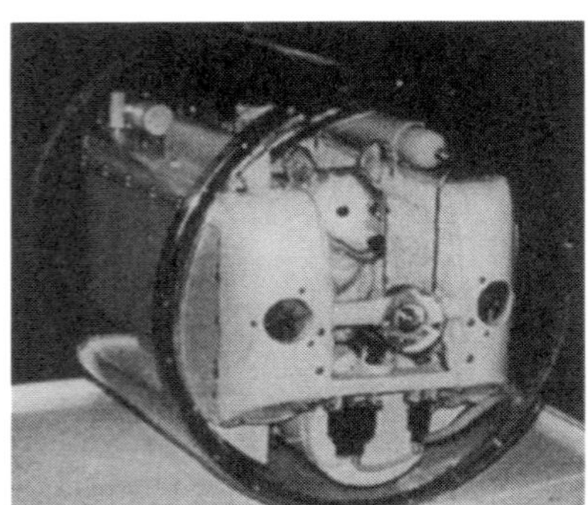

The challenges as well as barriers faced with providing health care in space are similar to those on earth, especially in the extreme environments. This is why analogs are important in evaluating approaches for addressing medical care in this regard. These challenges and barriers are highlighted in the section below.

Challenges and Barriers

There are many challenges and barriers to implementing telemedicine solutions. These challenges and barriers are highlighted in Table 1.

Table 1. Challenges and barriers facing implementation of telemedicine.

Challenges and Barriers
No immediate access to definitive care
Distance and geography
Limited communications
Limited diagnostic, treatment and pharmaceuticals
Language
Cultural diversity
Autonomy
Extreme conditions
Financial
Legislative policy
Socioeconomic / Political
Access
Technology (capabilities and availability)
Arrogance

This list of challenges and barriers is not reflective of one nation, one people, one race or one religion but effects all people, regardless of their locations. Each is explained herein.

No immediate return or access to definitive care. This is clear in the space program in that astronauts in low earth orbit cannot just depart their space station and land at a hospital. The same can be said about individuals who are located in places that are far removed from definitive care. This implies that distance is challenge. There are large populations around the world that are isolated by distance, which is not necessarily due to geography. It may in fact be merely the distance from one building to another in large city like New York or Moscow.

Communication is of course the key to any successful telemedicine activity [4]. However, communications can be limited in both time and rate or could be absent for periods of time. This illustrated in figure 2. This is an image of the orbital flight path of the Mir Space Station as seen at the Mission Control Center outside of Moscow, Russia. The only time there is communication is when the spacecraft is directly above the European / Asian landmass, which is highlighted by the black cloud.

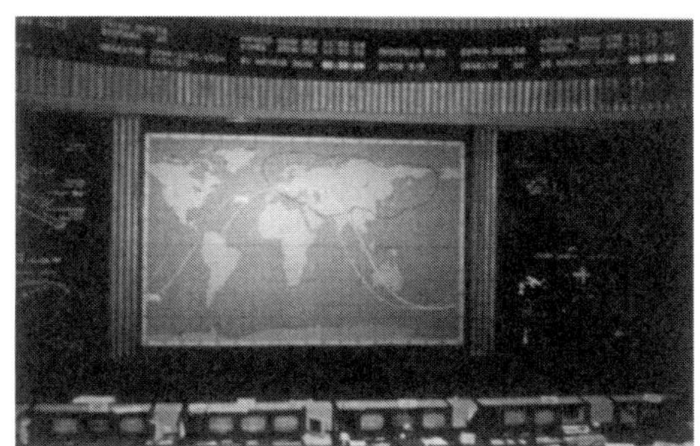

Figure 2. Mission Control Center in Kaliningrad, Russia

The rest of the time, there is no communications, which requires appropriate systems for autonomous operations. Communications can become an even greater issue when distances increase to the point that latency begins to approach several minutes. In fact, the communication delay between Earth and Mars is nearly 22 minutes one way. Those individuals who find themselves in a terrestrial location may also experience delays in communications or not have it at all. This again implies the need for limited autonomy. It is also important to note that telecommunications for medical care on space craft is low bandwidth. Not high speed or capacity at all.

Remote medical capabilities, whether in space or some outpost on earth, often times have limited diagnostic tools, limited treatment capabilities, and limited pharmaceuticals. This can be a significant challenge in addressing medical care because these limitations may in fact further exacerbate the situation. Limited resources can be of significant impact in implementing telemedicine.

Language and culture are of significant issue for many reasons. With regard to space flight, the nature of space exploration is now international by design. So the ability to communicate in a common language is important. This of course is not a great a challenge in space as it is on the ground. Depending on the country one fines themselves in, obtaining medical attention can be highly challenging because either the patient or the health care delivery system does not speak the same language, or there are nuances of language that can alter the treatment of the ability to treat. In some instances language can drive culture. Certainly, there are numerous cultural differences in the practice of medicine. This has been well known in the space program as well as in ground-based telemedicine projects such as the Space Bridge projects [5,6,7].

Additional challenges, which vary in importance and impact depending on the country or location within a geographic area, include financial, legislative, and policy. These are obviously tempered by socioeconomic and political positions. Funding can come from governments, foundations, philanthropists or the patients themselves. So the financial abilities to build and sustain telemedicine are a key challenge.

Legislation is important to telemedicine regardless of location. Each country's health department or ministry works to develop policies that address telemedicine. These policies can have an impact on the success of telemedicine implementation and ultimately access. Access can also be impacted by the capability and availability of technology. In some countries technology oozes out of the corner store. In other countries, it may take months to acquire what is needed to do the simplest of tasks.

With many of the challenges briefly addressed above, it is important to note, that arrogance can be the biggest challenge of all when it comes to telemedicine. This could be simply fear of change or fear of the unknown. The loss of control or the believe that they way it is done today is just fine and no change is needed. This of course has societal impact.

A Strategic Dilemma

As mention previously, humans exploration of space has utilize telemedicine since the late 1950s. Additionally, NASA conducted a number of ground-based test beds, which led to a need for a strategic plan to map its needs, requirements, and potential solutions. This strategic plan called for the creation of center of excellence with a focus on commercial partnerships. The result was establishment of the MITAC as a NASA Commercial Space Center.

MITAC was established at Yale University in 1997 and later moved to Virginia Commonwealth University in Richmond, VA in 1999. The MITAC has an objective of fostering telemedicine, telehealth, and medical informatics through the development of partnerships, which may be of direct benefit to NASA has a whole. There are three primary areas of interest. These include 1) Education, 2) Test Beds, and 3) Commercialization. The focus of this discussion will be primarily on the test beds.

Test Beds

Test beds provide unique opportunities to evaluate technologies and procedures for telemedicine applications. They are characterized by limited resources and can be used for validation. Test beds are also analogous to the environment of space. In all cases, these test beds are conducted using low bandwidth telecommunications. This has been previously highlighted above. MITAC's test beds that will be presented below include Mt. Everest, Devon Island, Russia, Kosova, Kenya, and Ecuador.

Mt. Everest

In 1998 and 1999, MITAC worked with several organizations in developing a monitoring system that could be used to access the location and physical condition of climbers on the ascent from base camp on Mt. Everest to the summit. Mt. Everest represents on of the most isolated places on Earth. Although there is a steady stream of climbers on the mountain in the spring, the conditions are severe and extreme. In 1995, several veteran mountain climbers lost their lives. Questions were raised about what could be done to make such outcomes different. Could technology be integrated in some way to monitor climbers position and their physiological status.

Working with Massachusetts Institute of Technology and others, MITAC developed a project that would permit climbers at Everest base camp to be monitored wirelessly by physicians at Yale University in New Haven, CT. A low bandwidth telecommunications system and suite of sensors was developed using commercial of the shelf equipment as well as custom designed devices. In 1998 and 1999, the telemedicine link between Everest base camp and Yale proved to be of great value. The concept of monitoring a physiological cipher was established and validated as a worthy step [8,9,10].

Devon Island

The lessons learned from the two Everest expeditions were applied at Devon Island in 2000. Devon Island, located in Northern Canada, is home to Haughton Crater. NASA and others have an interest in using this extreme site as an analog for future human missions to Mars. The terrain and extremes are similar to what might be seen on the Martian surface. In this test bed, MITAC outfitted a researcher with a wearable computer. A second researcher wore several sensors that were monitored wirelessly by the first researcher. All information collected was transmitted via the Internet to a MITAC server in Richmond. In addition, a delay of 22 minutes was factored in to simulate a mission on Mars. All information available on the second researcher, including vital signs and position, were ported to a Palm Pilot. This project validated the use of wireless technology and low bandwidth telecommunications as useful tool for telemedicine in extreme environments [11].

Kosova

During the Balkans war, the peoples of Kosova experienced severe health issues. Due in part to the war, but also because of the build up of refugees. In addition, medical schools in the Kosovar part of the former Yugoslavia were decimated. One of MITAC's faculty members, who is Albanian, has been very passionate about helping his homeland. In addition, NASA Headquarter asked MITAC what it might be able to due in support of the refugees. This prompted a quick design of a hub and spoke system. Although this plan was not implemented, there was a push to create the International Virtual E-Hospital. In addition, the Kosova Foundation for Medical Development was also established.

The challenge in Kosova was that of unique solutions for unique problems. Figure 3 illustrates simple kitchen utensils fashioned into surgical instruments. This device was used to support thoracic surgical intervention.

Figure 3. Simple kitchen utensils used as surgical instruments

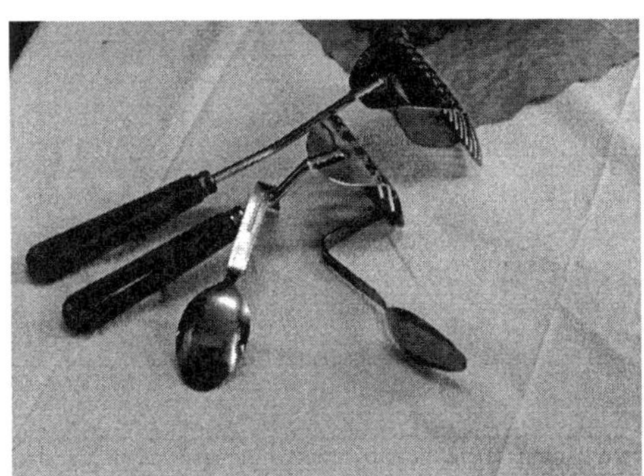

The solution in this environment is one of simplicity and cost. Highly effective telemedicine systems can be as simple as a digital camera and a low bandwidth Internet connection. For less than $1,000, telemedicine was conducted between Kosova and British medical forces quite effectively.

Since these events, there has been an inaugural opening of the Kosova Telemedicine Center at the Medical School of Prishtina. This facility implements many of the plans developed by MITAC.

Kenya

In 2000 and in 2002, MITAC provided telemedicine support for two different groups. The first was Operation Helping Hands and the second was a group of physicians and medical students. In both cases, telemedicine was implemented in support of medical relief missions. The effort in 2000 was supporting surgical cases. In this test bed, telemedicine was used for prescreening of surgical cases. One such case involved a male patient who had received an injury to his forearm from an alligator. Surgeons in Richmond used telemedicine to manage this case prior to traveling to Kenya to perform the surgery. Telecommunications between rural sites in Kenya and Richmond was accomplished using an Inmarsat satellite phone linked to mobile, rapidly deployable telemedicine unit.

The work in 2002, was focused on infectious disease. Physicians, who traveled to Kenya from Richmond, remained in communication with Richmond through a satellite phone. Since the majority of work was done in remote areas, power for the computers, satellite phones, and personal digital assistants was provided by a deployable solar power grid, which was connected to a car battery.

Kenya was characterized by poor infrastructure and limited access to knowledge bases. Yet there were modern operating rooms available. Pre-planning, needs assessment, and expectation of the unexpected were key to these test beds.

Ecuador

Ecuador has many different areas where telemedicine has been evaluated and validated. These range from rural, jungle areas accessible by poor dirt roads to areas that are only accessible by small plane or boat. This test bed has provided unique opportunities because of the wide range of challenges. These include delivering health care using mobile facilities, low bandwidth communications – such HF radio, and interaction in extremely remote regions.

Telemedicine in Ecuador has included many first, including the first transmission of images for anatomical confirmation, tele-anethesia, and support of pre-surgical screening [12,13].

Summary

These test beds have provided a unique opportunity to evaluate and validate telemedicine technologies in extreme environments. These environments are similar in many ways to what might be observed in space. These then are considered effective analogs for space flight. Many problems require complex solutions but there are many problems that can be solved with simple solutions. For additional information on MITAC or other programs, please visit www.meditac.com.

References

[1] Doarn CR, Lavrentyev V, Orlov OI, Grigoriev A, Nicogossian AE, Ferguson EW, Merrell RC. Evolution of telemedicine in Russia: Influences from the space program. A ten-year summary. Telemed J E-Health 9(1): – At Press

[2] Lugg D, Shepanek M. Space analogue studies in Antarctica. Acta Astronaut, 44(7-12):693-699, 1999

[3] Hyer RN. Telemedical experience at an Antarctic station. J Telemed Telecare 5(Suppl 1):S87-89. 1999

[4] Mandil SH. Telematics in Health Care in Developing Countries. J Med Sys 19(2):195-203, 1995

[5] Doarn CR, Nicogossian AE, Merrell RC. Application of Telemedicine in the United States Space Program. Telemed J, 4(1):19-30. 1998

[6] Angood PB, Doarn CR, Holaday L, Nicogossian AE, Merrell RC. The Spacebridge to Russia Project: Internet-Based Telemedicine. Telemed J, 4(4):305-11. 1999

[7] Doarn CR, Nicogossian AE, Merrell RC. Application of Telemedicine in the United States Space Program. Telemed J, 4(1):19-30. 1998

[8] Angood PB, Satava R, Doarn C, Merrell R, and E3 Group. Telemedicine at the top of the world; the 1998-1999 Everest Extreme Expedition. Telemed J and e-Health, 6(3):315-25, 2001

[9] Satava RM, Angood PB, Harnett B, Macedonia C, and Merrell RC. The physiological cipher at altitude: telemedicine and real-time monitoring of climbers on Mount Everest. Telemed J and e-Health, 6(3):303-13, 2001

[10] Harnett, BM, Satava S, Angood P, Merriam NR, Doarn CR, Merrell RC. The Benefits of Integrating Internet Technology with Standard Communications for Telemedicine in Extreme Environments Aviat Space Environ Med 2001; 72:1132-7

[11] Harnett BM, Doarn CR, Russell KM, Kapoor V, Merriam NR, Merrell RC. Wireless Telemetry and Internet Technologies for Medical Management: A Martian Analogy. Aviat Space Environ Med. 72(12):1125-1131. 2001.

[12] Praba-Egge A, Hummel R, Stewart N, Doarn CR, Merrell RC. Remote telemedicine services by high frequency radio link. J Clin Eng 28(1):37-42. 2003 – At Press.

[13] Doarn CR, Fitzgerald S, Rodas E, Harnett B, Merrell RC. Telemedicine to Integrate Intermittent Surgical Services in to Primary Care. Telemed J E-Health, 8(1):131-137, 2002.

Address for correspondence

Charles R. Doarn, MBA
Executive Director
Medical Informatics and Technology Applications Consortium
Assistant Professor
Department of Surgery
Virginia Commonwealth University
PO Box 980480, Richmond, VA 23298-0480, USA
phone: +1 (804) 827-1022
fax: +1 (804) 827-1029
e.mail: crdoarn@hsc.vcu.edu

Development of a Robotic Navigation and Fracture Fixation System

BERND FUECHTMEIER[1], STEFAN EGERSDOERFER[2],
GEORG TUMA[3], GERIT J. MONKMAN[2], MICHAEL NERLICH[1]

[1]*Department of Trauma Surgery, University of Regensburg,
Franz-Josef-Strauss Allee 11, 93053 Regensburg, Germany*
[2]*Fachhochschule Regensburg - University of Applied Sciences, Fachbereich,
Elektrotechnik, Prüfeninger Strasse 58, 93049 Regensburg, Germany*
[3]*Brainlab AG, Ammerthalstrasse 8, 85551 München/Heimstetten*

Abstract. The use of robotics in surgery is nothing new. However, there are areas of surgery, such as in fracture fixation, where robots have yet to be implemented. This paper considers the choice of robot, gripper and ancillary equipment together with navigation systems necessary for their application.

Hitherto robots have seen operation in surgery only in cases where relatively low manipulation forces are required. Nothing yet exists with the capability of handling forces in excess of 200 Newton as would be required in the above scenario. Another encumbrance to robots which are already in medical use is the difficulty in programming. Unfortunately most of these robots are programmed by specialists for a particular application. However, there exists a number of robot programming languages, like Unimation VA-LII (recently superceded by Stäubli V+), which do not require specialist knowledge. The application of industrial robots to the „heavier" side of modern surgery is without doubt technically realisable. The remainder of this research project aims to determine exactly which robots and what ancilliary equipment are needed and then to implement them, first on plastic models and later on cadavers. A second phase is expected to deal with type approval and a final third phase with operations on live patients.

Introduction

The repair of broken limbs by surgery often necessitates the application of considerable force in order to displace one or both ends of a broken bone against the natural forces of muscle and tendon. A typical situation is a fractured femur or fibula in which both ends lay beside one another after the muscles have relaxed. These parts of the bone must then be pulled away from one another and held stationary before being precisely positioned end to end to allow correct mending. Conventionally this is carried out by surgeons and medical staff with the help of occasional x-ray images for navigation purposes. There is always the danger of physical overshoot - resulting in unnecessary muscle, tissue and ligament strain during the manipulation process and excessive x-ray exposure is desirable for neither patient nor medical staff. Furthermore, due to the large necessary holding forces, exact "first time" positioning is virtually impossible. What is needed is an automated system whereby the fracture ends of the bone may be precisely positioned without overshoot and held in place as long as necessary before being brought together in exactly the correct position without the necessity for multiple docking attempts. Preliminary measurements made during operations with single axis force sensors have shown that forces up to around 260 Newtons are required.

Robotics

Hitherto robots have been used during surgery only in cases where relatively low manipulation forces are required such as the positioning of endoscopes [1], small surgical instruments in keyhole or neurosurgery [2] or fibre optics in the case of laser surgery [3]. Recently, some advances have been made in the use of hexapod robots in bone machining [4] and some robots have been used for the positioning of implants [5], but nothing yet exists with the capability of handling forces in excess of 200 Newton as would be required in the above scenario. Another encumbrance to robots which are already in medical use is the difficulty in programming. Surgeons often complain that using the robot extends, rather than reduces, the time needed to complete surgery. Table 1 shows a number of robots which are already approved for medical use, together with their relative load capabilities and programming language formats.

Table 1. Medically approved robots

Manufacturer	Robot Type	Maximum load	Applications
orto-MARQUET (D)	CASPAR	60 N	orthopaedic
Zeiss (D)	Hexapod	200 N	orthopaedic
Armstrong Healthcare Ltd. (UK)	EndoAssist	Endoscopic instruments	MIS
Computer Motion (US)	ZEUS	Endoscopic instruments	MIS
Intuitive Surgical Inc. (US)	Da Vinci	Endoscopic instruments	MIS
Integrated Surgical Systems (US)	NeuroMate	Endoscopic instruments	MIS
Computer Motion (US)	AESOP	Endoscopic instruments	MIS
ISS Inc./SelMcKenzie (US)	RoboDoc	150 N	Hip arthroplasty
Pyxis (US)	Helpmate	Mobile robot	Delivery

The robots in table 1 are medically approved in at least one country, few if any, are capable of handling the large loads necessary in fracture fixation.

Many industrial robots capable of fulfilling these needs are already commercially available. Manipulation forces of 500 Newton is just a minimal force for a typical welding robot used in automobile manufacturing.

Unfortunately, most of these robots are programmed by specialists for a particular application, which will run without modification for several months. In fact, one of the main problems resulting from the implementation of robots in non-traditional robotic areas is that the manufacturers try to develop a programming system so simple that it becomes too cumbersome for all but the simplest of functions. However, there exists a number of robot programming languages, like Unimation VALII (recently superceded by Stäubli V+), which do not require specialist knowledge beyond that of which the average surgeon is more than capable [6]. Table 2 lists a number (many more are also commercially available) of industrial robots potentially capable of being used in fracture fixation.

Table 2. Standard industrial robots

Manufacturer	Type	Weight	Maximum load	Prog. Language	Structure
ASEA	IRB-4400/30	940 kg	300 N	RAPID	Compiler
	IRB-4400/60	1019 kg	600 N	RAPID	Compiler
Fanuc	M-16i	370 kg	160 N	KAREL	Interpreter
	M-710i	600 kg	450 N	KAREL	Interpreter
	M-710w	820 kg	700 N	KAREL	Interpreter
Kuka	KR15	875 kg	150 N	SoftPLC/KRL	Compiler
	KR30	867 kg	300 N	SoftPLC/KRL	Compiler
	KR45	875 kg	450 N	SoftPLC/KRL	Compiler
	KR60	875 kg	600 N	SoftPLC/KRL	Compiler
Stäubli	RX130	220 kg	240 N	V+	Interpreter
	RX170	730 kg	600 N	V+	Interpreter

Most of the robots listed in table 2, particularly those from ASEA and Kuka, are relatively heavy. The lighter models often lack the strength needed for the task, though the Stäubli RX130 would be on the border of its capabilities. Fanuc robots are problematic in that Fanuc's company policy prohibits them from involvement in military or medical robotics.

As outlined by Flury and co-workers [2], among others, there are many other reasons why most industrial robots cannot be used for medical purposes as they stand. Though most of the robots in table 2 are physically capable of handling the loads required, to meet type approval certain modifications must be made:

1. Most industrial robots are capable of velocities in excess of 2 m/s. This is dangerously fast in medical situations where speeds in the region of 0.1 m/s and less are more reasonable. Some form of hardware (not just software) speed limit must be incorporated. This could by achieved mechanically by using only large gear ratio harmonic drives [7], or by limiting the speed of synchronous motors electrically by sharp roll-off low pass filtering the drive signals.

2.In an emergency situation it must be possible for the surgeon to manually move the robot arm temporarily away from the patient and operating area. This must also be possible with the robot switched of, i.e. in the event of a power failure. Many robots do incorporate such a facility, such as air brakes which may be switched out pneumatically by pressing a suitably located button.

3.It is also preferred that the robot is portable. That is, mounted on a movable platform which may be easily transferred from one operating theatre to another. This can place limits on the weight of the robot or demands on the capabilities of the vehicle on which it is mounted. In fact, two of the smaller robots listed in table 2, namely the Fanuc M-16i and the Kuka KR15, are unlikely to meet the payload requirements. However, they clearly show how the overall weight of a given robot reduces with reduced payload capability - over-dimensioned robots are clearly to be avoided! Vehicular systems based on fork-lift truck technology are commercially available [8]. Some are also type approved for use in hospitals [9]. The necessary modifications needed for robot transport purposes are technically trivial.

None of the above problems are insurmountable. However, most constitute some degree of modification to existing designs to meet DIN/EN60601 compliance [10].

Of the four categories of robot gripper (impactive, ingressive, astrictive and contigutive) only impactive types are of real relevance. That the gripper must prehend the carbon fibre shaft which connects and supports the bone securing pins, rather than the patients limbs, is of advantage.

Pneumatically driven impactive grippers (Figure 1) intended for industrial use are more than adequate for this task. Suitable gripper fingers will be designed for this purpose. In addition, it may be desirable to modify the surface of the shaft to prevent slippage during manipulation. However, polygonal shaft cross-sections may have to be avoided owing to the danger of sudden movements as the gipper and shaft mechanically mate together.

Figure 1. Pneumatically driven impactive robot gripper

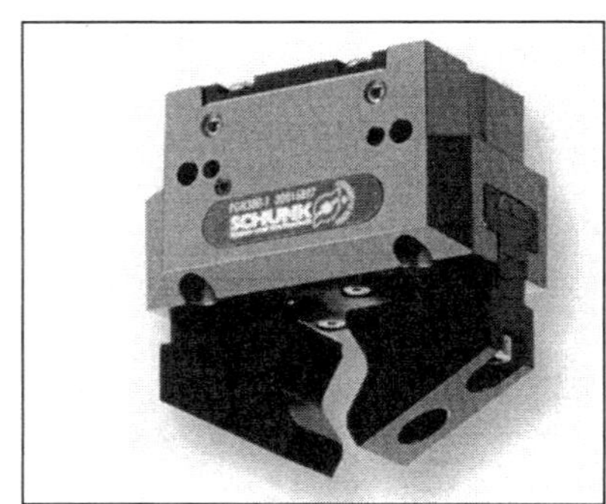

This problem may be reduced to some extent by using a degree of mechanical compliance. Remote Centre Compliance (RCC) units can be inserted between the robot wrist and the gripper [6]. These may be passive or active and can include a degree of instrumentation for force and torque measurements.

Figure 2. Typical Remote Centre Compliance (RCC) mechanism [JR3]

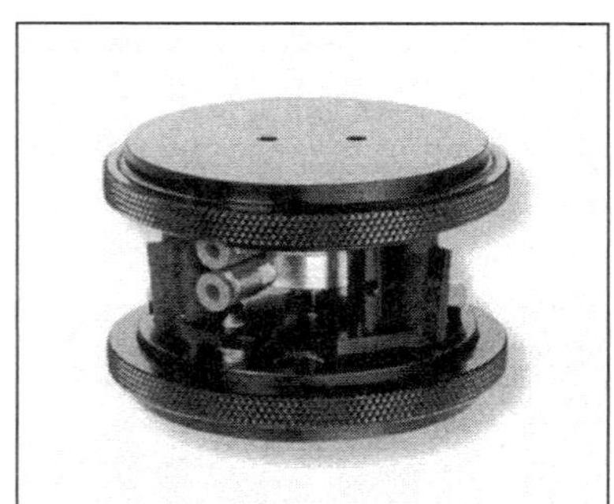

During operation of the robot, it will be necessary to constantly monitor force and torque applied to the patient via the gripper. In addition to instrumented RCCs, discrete force/torque sensor units are commercially available (Table 3) and can, like the RCC, be fitted between the robot wrist and the gripper.

Table 3. Commercially available force/torque sensors

Manufacturer	Type	Integrated Force/Torque Sensor	Kinaesthetic Force/Torque Feedback
ASEA	IRB-4400/30	ATI (Schunk)	
	IRB-4400/60	ATI (Schunk)	
Fanuc	M-16i	Fanuc	
	M-710i	Fanuc	
	M-710w	Fanuc	
Kuka	KR15	JR3/ATI/DLR/HBM	Amatec
	KR30	JR3/ATI/DLR/HBM	Amatec
	KR45	JR3/ATI/DLR/HBM	Amatec
	KR60	JR3/ATI/DLR/HBM	Amatec
Stäubli	RX130	JR3	
	RX170	JR3	

Kinaesthetic feedback (reflected force feedback) is often preferred by surgeons because they get a feeling for the real situation. This allows a robot to be roughly positioned by simple teleoperation, the force feedback being useful in guiding the surgeon and preventing excess force being delivered. Finer positioning can then be carried out under program control with force and torque feedback being used to stop the robot, or reverse its movement, in the event of a predetermined force threshold being reached.

Navigation Systems

Passive and/or offline planning and navigation systems are already highly developed, as in Pathfinder from Armstrong Healthcare or the CASPAR system from URS [URS]. However, for robotic guidance during trauma surgery, it is necessary for the robot to obtain knowledge about the actual position of the bone fractures during the operation. In other words, the robot has to be able to "see" what even the surgeon can only see by continuously radiating the patient and himself with X-rays.

These "seeing-eyes" are represented by Brainlab's VectorVision® Navigation System - an infrared camera detects the position of the patient's broken bones and the position of the image itensifier (standard c-arm). Acquiring these images and following the surgeons planning of the target bone position, the system can calculate and visualize the necessary kinematic transformations (translation and rotation) needed to achieve a correct bone alignment. X-ray data received from the C-arm provides a Graphical User Interface for planning and sends the movement data to the Robot. Additional tools - driven freehand by the surgeon or automatically by the robot - can be integrated and visualized in virtual reality (Figure 3). To capture the position and track the movement of patients anatomy or surgical tools the surgeon has to attach reflecting coordinate systems ("rigid body") to the bony structures and to the instruments (or e.g. the robot arm).

Figure 3. Basic Principle of Robot Assisted Trauma Surgery

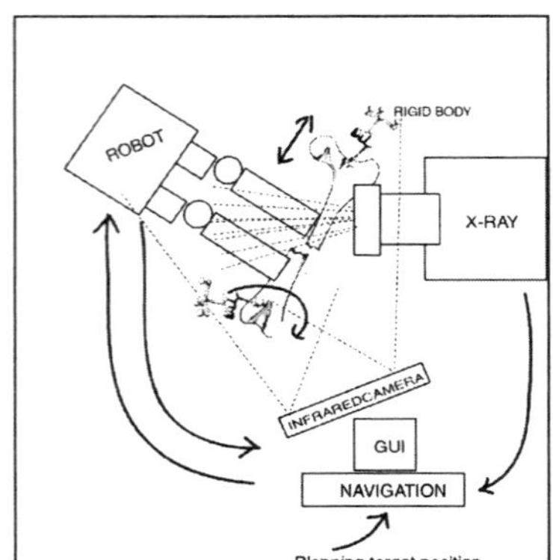

The c-arm visualizes the position of the fragments (in different view-angles) inside the patients body.

The navigation systems camera captures the X-rays projection matrix and the "rigid bodies" fixed to the bone in order to continuously track position changes.

The surgeon plans the target position of the bone alignment at the navigation system. This produces the necessary data to allow the robot to align the bone fragments in the planned manner (Figure 4).

Figure 4. Flowchart of robotic components

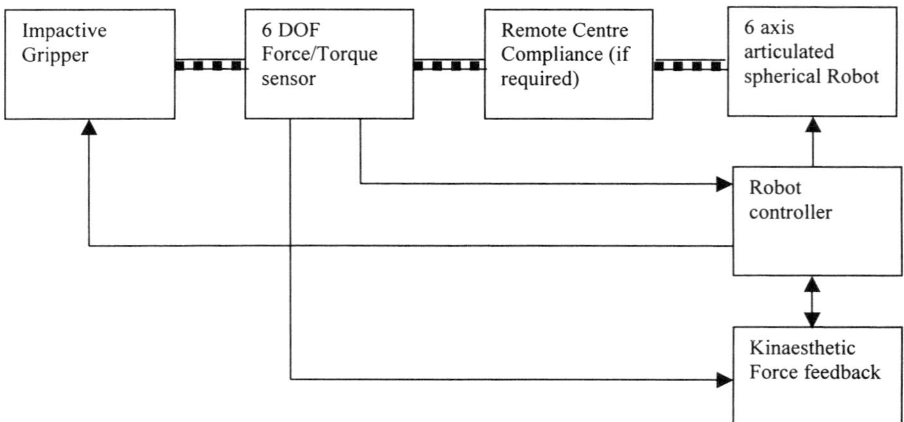

Conclusions

The application of industrial robots to the "heavier" side of modern surgery is without doubt technically realisable. The remainder of this research project aims to determine exactly which robots and what ancilliary equipment are needed and then to implement them, first on plastic models and later on cadavers. A second phase is expected to deal with type approval and a final third phase with surgery on live patients.

References

[1]　Mueglitz. J, G. Kunad, P. Dautzenberg, B. Neisius & R. Trapp - Kinematic Problems of Manipulators for Minimal Invasive Surgery - Endoscopic Surgery, pp 160-164. - Georg Thieme Verlag, Stuttgart, 1993.

[2]　Flury. P, P. Lopez, D. Glauser, N. Villotte & C.W. Burckhardt - MINERVA, a robot dedicated to neurosurgeryl operations - Proceedings 23rd Int. Symposium on Robotics (ISR '92). pp 729-733 - Barcelona, October 1992.

[3]　Monkman. G.J. - New technique kills "inoperable" tumours - Biophotonics International - pp. 20-21, Laurin Pubs., May/June 1996.

[4]　Wapler. J., Th. Weisener, A. Hiller - Hexapod-Robot System for Precision Surgery - Proceedings 29th Int. Symposium on Robotics (ISR '98) - April 1998.

[5]　Pransky. J. - Surgeons realisations of RoboDoc - Industrial Robot No. 25, pp105-108 - MCB Press,1998.

[6]　McKerrow. P.J. - Introduction to Robotics - Addison-Wesley, 1991.

[7]　Harmonic Drive - Applications Handbook - Version 2, Harmonic Drive, Limburg 1992.

[8]　Crown Gabelstapler GmbH - Hahnenbalz 35, 90411 Nürnberg.

[9]　NDC - Netzler & Dahlgren Co. AB, SE-429 80 SÄRÖ, Schweden.

[10]　VDE 0750 – DIN/EN 60601 Medizinische elektrische Geräte – VDE Vorschriftenwerk, 1993.

Acknowledgements

The authors would like to gratefully acknowledge the financial support of the DFG, close cooperation offered by the company Brainlab and the kind assistance and advice from Prof. Dr.-Ing. Gerd Hirzinger and Dipl.-Ing. Ulrich Hagn of DLR.

Address for correspondence

Bernd Fuechtmeier, MD
Department of Trauma Surgery
University of Regensburg
93042 Regensburg, Germany
phone: +49 941 944 0
fax:　　+49 941 944 6806
e.mail: bernd.fuechtmeier@klinik.uni-regensburg.de

Integration of Health Telematics into Medical Practice
M. Nerlich and U. Schaechinger (Eds.)
IOS Press, 2003

A Readiness Model for Telehealth
Is it possible to Pre-Determine How Prepared Communities are to Implement Telehealth?

PENNY JENNETT[1], JOANNA BATES[2], THERESA HEALY[3],
KENDALL HO[4], ARMINEE KAZANJIAN[2], ROBERT WOOLLARD[2],
ANDORA JACKSON[1], SUSAN HAYDT[5]

[1] *Health Telematics Unit (HTU), University of Calgary, Calgary, Alberta, Canada*
[2] *Faculty of Medicine, University of British Columbia, Vancouver, B.C., Canada*
[3] *Environmental Planning, University of Northern British Columbia,*
Prince George, B.C., Canada
[4] *Continuing Medical Education, University of British Columbia, Vancouver, B.C., Canada*
[5] *Department of Sociology, University of Calgary, Calgary Alberta, Canada*

Abstract. Telehealth "readiness" can be defined as the degree to which users, health care organizations, and the health system itself are prepared to participate and succeed in its application. This project developed a readiness model for rural/remote locations in Canada. Specifically defined groups or communities with shared characteristics within a rural geographical community (i.e. practitioners, patients, the public, and health care organizations) participated in key informant interviews, awareness sessions, focus groups, and face-to-face interviews. The data were examined and organized keeping in mind Weiss' Program's Theory of Change. This approach allowed concrete and abstract factors to be considered. The model that emerged suggests that there are four types of readiness for each of the defined communities: core, engagement, structural, and non-readiness. The "communities" share some readiness factors and risks, but also exhibit unique elements. This finding is critical to acknowledge when the goal is to implement a useful, effective, and sustainable telehealth system within remote settings. Study results hold a key to understanding why technology systems have failed in the past, in spite of dedicating considerable human and financial resources towards their implementation. Notations of these findings will be helpful in future telehealth implementations within rural and isolated areas.

Purpose and Rationale

Over 30% of the Canadian population resides in rural or remote areas. Such populations are at risk with respect to health status, quality care, and access [1]. Telehealth has the potential to improve the access and quality of health care in rural/remote communities. Failure rates of 30% and greater are associated with large-scale Information Technology (IT) projects [2,3,4]. Considering the substantial initial investment in IT to establish telehealth, it would be more efficient to determine ahead of time whether a community is ready for its implementation. This project developed a telehealth "readiness" model for rural/remote locations in Canada. It defined the essence of "readiness" for rural/remote communities.

Definitions and Concepts

Readiness
- the "cognitive precursor to the behaviors of either resistance to, or support for, a change effort" [5]
- the initial and essential step in the change process [6,7,8,9,19]
- the degree to which a community is prepared to participate and succeed in telehealth [11]
Communities
- include the rural/remote geographical communities
- groups within the overall community with shared characteristics (patients who share a common problem, health providers, organizations, and members of the public) [12]
Rural
- Health Canada divides rural areas into rural metro-adjacent, rural heartlands, and rural northern/remote [13]

Methods

The data collection strategy was to approach the specially defined communities within the rural geographical communities (i.e. the health care providers, the patients, the public, and health care organizations). Experts participated in sixteen key informant audio-taped telephone interviews. There were two community awareness sessions, followed by five audio-taped focus groups (5-8 participants in each), and two in-depth interviews with community physicians. The data approach and analysis are illustrated in Figure 1.

Figure 1. Data Approach & Analysis [14,15,16]

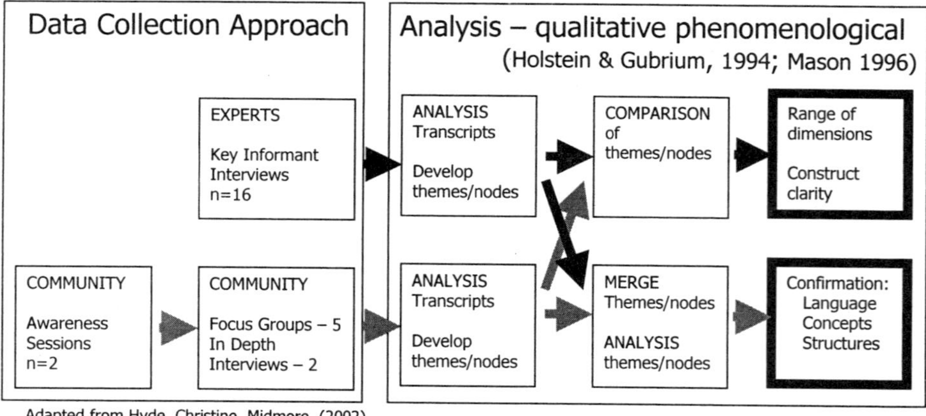

The data were examined and organized in keeping with Weiss' Program's Theory of Change [17]. This approach allows tangible and less tangible factors to be considered. Program Theory and Implementation Theory are combined to produce the program's theory of change.

Program Theory looks at the intangible factors that will affect telehealth implementation and can be applied at any time before, during, or after implementation. These intangible factors are influenced by:
- Attitudes – e.g. fears, willingness to take a risk, and willingness to try new things
- Cultural factors - e.g. expectations around gender roles and the socioeconomic status of the people involved
- Knowledge/skills – e.g. awareness of the potential of telehealth and ability to use the equipment
- Relationships between/within communities – e.g. cooperation, consulting with communities to determine their needs, organizations granting users autonomy over the use of equipment, and allowing for creativity in determining other uses.

Implementation Theory gives the steps identified by key informants to implement a successful telehealth service. The first step is to determine the needs of a given community. Secondly, a telehealth application must be decided upon, such as who will use it where, when, and for what purpose. To build a telehealth infrastructure is the third step; ensuring that the funding, technology, personnel, management, policies, and procedures are in place. Fourthly, the implementation of telehealth needs to fulfill the expected outcomes. For instance telehealth should address the identified needs of the community, and be used once it is implemented. The final step is to make sure that the service is sustained.

Results

The patient, practitioner, organizational, and public communities shared some factors of readiness, but also exhibited unique elements. Types of "readiness" in each of these communities could be divided into *core*, *engagement*, and *structural* readiness. *Core* readiness was when there was an identification of a need and a desire for change. This was identified as a type of readiness in all of the "communities". The current state of health care was considered inadequate and the remote location was the source of many health care needs.

The *engagement* level of readiness could be described as questioning and assessing risks. Examples of factors found within the *engagement* type of readiness within the patient and practitioner communities are outlined in Table 1.

Table 1. Examples of Factors within the Engagement "Type"

Patient	Practitioner
Knowledge about what exactly telehealth is	Innovators; champions
Knowledge about benefits	Sense of curiosity
Fear of damaging equipment	Peer influence
Gender	Evidence of utility
Privacy concerns	Inter-group cooperation (practitioner and other domains)
Availability/reliability of content that fits rural culture	
Address concerns about telehealth replacing current services	Intra-group cooperation (between practitioners)
	Communication
Sense of ownership	Openness; respect for others
	Willingness to make initial investment in time

Structural readiness included building efficient structures and supports

There were many questions in the area of structural readiness. Sufficient people, technical structures, and training available were stated requirements of all "communities". People's perception of the structure of telehealth influenced their level of engagement readiness.

Non-readiness of a community was identified when a community was unable to recognize that telehealth could assist with its health and healthcare needs. The data indicated that there were some examples of non-readiness in the communities [18].

Perceived Risks in Telehealth & Proposed Solutions

Communities weighed the risks that they felt in telehealth against the benefits they felt it would bring. Some of the perceived risks overlap between "communities" and some are unique to a particular "community". For example, one concern within the Patient Community was their lack of stated technical skills, and the impact that might have on a patient's ability to successfully access and use telehealth. A response to this would be to offer education to patients in home-based applications; the supplying organization could be responsible for technical support. Further, the technology could be simplified by using touch screens instead of mouse/keyboard driven computers, or by using the telephone instead of a computer.

Another example of an apprehension that practitioners shared was that telehealth might provide information that was incorrect or inapplicable to their practice. A possible solution for this concern would be to confer with practitioners about the information provided, so that they would be more confident in its reliability and applicability. Practitioners could be actively involved in designing applications, for instance deciding what Continuing Medical Education (CME) topics would be provided. Further concerns and potential solutions to address readiness challenges can be found in Jennett et al., 2003 [18].

Conclusions and Summary

As "readiness" for telehealth is a key prerequisite to successful implementation, it is mandatory that stakeholders within telehealth begin to understand its complex and ubiquitous nature. This study examined the essence of readiness as it applies to rural/remote settings. It found four types of readiness and multiple factors within each type. Project findings also note that readiness can vary between key defined communities (e.g. public, patient, practitioner and organization). Risks for telehealth implementation, along with solutions for such concerns, were outlined. The knowledge gained from this study will be helpful for rural/remote communities as they consider or implement telehealth.

References

[1]   Health Canada. *Towards a Healthy Future: Second Report on the Health of Canadians.* Federal, Provincial and Territorial Advisory Committee on Population Health, 1999 (Cat. No. H39-468/1999E).

[2]   Dowling, A.F. Do hospital staff interfere with computer system implementation? *Health Care Management Review* 1980;5: 23-32.

[3]   Lyytien, K., & Hirschheim, R. (1987). Information system failure - a survey and classification of empirical literature. *Oxford Surveys in Information Technology* 1987;4: 257-309.

[4]   More, E. Information systems: People issues. *Journal of Information Sciences* 1990;16:311-320.

[5]   Armenakis, A.A., Harris, S.G., & Mossholder, K.W. Creating readiness for organizational change. *Human Relations* 1993;46 (6): 681-703.

[6]   Lewin, K. Frontiers in group dynamics. *Human Relations* 1947; 1: 5-41.
[7]   Lewin, K. *Field theory in social science*. New York: Harper and Row, 1951
[8]   Coch & French. Overcoming resistance to change. *Human Relations* 1948; 1: 512-532.
[9]   Prochaska, J.O. & DiClemente, C.C. Transtheoretical therapy: Toward a more integrative model of change. *Psychotherapy: Theory, Research, and Practice* 1982; 19: 275-288.
[10] Rogers, E.M. *Diffusions of innovations* (3rd ed.). New York: Free Press, 1983.
[11] Information Technologies Group, Center for International Development at Harvard University, (2002). *Readiness for the Networked World: A Guide for Developing Countries*. Accessed at http://www.readinessguide.org/ on February 26, 2002.
[12] Taggart, W.H.J. *Enablement and the Community: A Policy Approach for the Future*. Ottawa, ON: Canada Mortgage and Housing Corporation, 1997.
[13] Lyons, R., & Gardner, P., (Nov. 2001). Building a Strong Foundation for Rural and Remote Health Research in Canada. *St. John's Rural Health Research Forum Summary Notes*, St. John's, Newfoundland, September 7-9, 2001. Accessed at http://www.cihr.ca/news/reports_proceedings/report_e.shtml on January 15, 2002.
[14] Hyde, T., Christie, M., Midmore, P. (2001). Introducing rigour into the design and development of choice experiment survey instruments. *Choice Experiments Conference 2001 Proceedings*. Online www.irs.aber.ac.uk/mec/Ceconf.htm.
[15] Holstein, J.A. & Gubrium, J.F. (1994). Phenomenology, ethnomethodology, and interpretive practice. In N.K. Denzin & Y.S. Lincoln (Eds.), *Handbook of qualitative methods*. Thousand Oaks, CA: Sage Publications.
[16] Mason, J. 1996. *Qualitative Researching.* Thousand Oaks, CA: Sage Publications.
[17] Weiss, C. "Understanding the Program" in *Evaluation: Methods for Studying Programs and Policies* (2nd ed.) Upper Saddle River, N.J.: Prentice Hall, 1998.
[18] Jennett, P.; Jackson, A.; Healy, T.; Ho, K.; Kazanjian, A.; Woollard, R.; Haydt, S.; Bates, J. A Study of Telehealth Readiness in Rural Communities. *Journal of Telemedicine and Telecare* 2003 (in press).

Acknowledgements

Local Research Assistants:
- Gilat Linn – University of British Columbia
- Christina McLennan – University of Northern British Columbia
Community Members and Volunteers
Key Informants
Funding Sources:
- CANARIE
- Health Canada
Manuscript Preparation:
- Marilyn Letts

Address for Correspondence

Dr. Penny Jennett
Professor, Faculty of Medicine, Head, Health Telematics Unit
University of Calgary
G204 Health Sciences Centre
3330 Hospital Drive NW,
Calgary, Alberta, Canada, T2N 4N1
phone: (403) 220 6845
fax::   (403) 270 8025
e.mail: jennett@ucalgary.ca

An Automated Diagnostic System for Tubular Carcinoma of the Breast – An Overview of Approach and Considerations

F. JOEL W-M. LEONG[1], JAMES O'D. McGEE[2]

[1]Oxford University Nuffield Department of Clinical Laboratory Sciences, John Radcliffe Hospital, Oxford OX3 9DU, United Kingdom
[2]Oxford University Nuffield Department of Medicine, John Radcliffe Hospital, Oxford OX3 9DU, United Kingdom

Abstract. A computer-based automated histopathology recognition system was developed to distinguish benign from malignant lesions. Tubular carcinoma of the breast, which has several reactive and neoplastic mimics, was selected as a model. Archival stained tumour sections from the United Kingdom National External Quality Assurance Scheme for breast pathology and supplementary material from external pathologists formed the study population. A diagnostic process similar to that employed by the histopathologist was adopted, viz, low-power feature extraction and analysis by cluster/glandular groupings followed by high-power confirmation. To circumvent problems of stain variability, greyscale quantisation of images was achieved through Karhunen-Loeve transformation with results suggesting that histological stains provide information primarily through contrast and not colour. Mean nearest neighbour and variance of cell nuclei distances were found to be 100% effective in distinguishing images which contained diffuse tumour, and no clustering. Gaussian smoothing followed by minimum variance quantisation allowed segmentation of gland clusters. Perona-Malik nonlinear diffusion filter employed prior to intensity thresholding and morphological filtering was 92% (7330/7973) effective in segmenting individual glands. In a set of 62 benign and 52 malignant gland clusters, the features found to discriminate tubular carcinoma from benign conditions included >20% of glands with sharp-angled edge, cluster area >150,000 pixels, ratio total gland area:total cluster area <0.14, >60 glands per cluster and the ratio average malignant gland area:benign gland area <0.5. Suspicious clusters were subjected to high-power feature analysis for nuclear morphology, nucleoli detection and basement membrane assessment. Watershed thresholding achieved nuclear segmentation and nuclear area >1.3x mean benign nuclear area was found to have a malignant likelihood ratio of 14.5. Progressive thresholding was used to detect nucleoli. Basement membrane was accentuated by colour segmentation and demonstrated 0.96 sensitivity, 0.89 specificity and 0.92 positive predictive value for distinguishing malignancy.

Introduction

The application of image processing in pathology, in the broadest sense, extends back as far as the 1970s. Much of this work involved individual cell analysis, that is, cytology. Bacus et al. 1976 [1] examined 325 blood film erythrocytes from 11 different classes under an oil immersion (100x) objective in an attempt to determine the best criteria to separate them into diagnostic subgroups. Details on the method of digitisation and image size were not provided. Recognising variations in size and shape of red blood cells has clinical utility in the diagnosis of different types of anaemia. They found that five features – size, roundness, spicularity, eccentricity and central gray level distribution allowed separation of erythrocytes into six classes – macrocyte, normocyte, spiculed (schistocyte, acanthocyte, Burr cell), microcyte (microcyte, spherocyte), oblong (elliptocyte, sickle cell, pencil form) and target. This work probably laid the foundation for the current range automated haematological blood film analysers that are a common and expected part of modern medical practice.

To date, much work in the area of automated diagnostic systems in histopathology has originated from Peter Bartels, in Arizona [2-23]. The work presented here is different both in its approach and the organ studied. Bartels' group has a long history of developing systems for automated diagnostic histopathology in the areas of prostatic intraepithelial neoplasia [18,19,21], prostatic carcinoma [13,15,16,22,24], thyroid disease [4,9], and colorectal carcinoma [5,9,25] although concrete data validating the accuracy of automated diagnosis against human interpretation has been less forthcoming.

Other research has been more specialised and image analysis in histopathology has largely been manually implemented or at most executed in a semi-automated manner. Textural analysis has been used in the nuclear grading of prostatic lesions [18,19,26-28], adrenal cortical carcinomas [29], brain tumors [30,31], in the identification of malignant colonic mucosa [32] and the grading of breast cancer [33-35]. Recently, wavelets have been used to extract parameters for the description of chromatin texture in the cytological diagnosis and grading of breast cancer [36,37].

Bayesian Belief Networks have been used for computer-aided diagnosis in prostatic pathology [38,39] and breast fine needle aspiration biopsies [40,41]. Keenan et al. [42] developed an automated machine vision system for histological grading of cervical intraepithelial neoplasia (CIN). Using a Delaunay triangulation mesh create from the centre of each epithelial cell nucleus, they measured number of physical parameters such as nuclear area, nuclear to cytoplasmic ratio, and location within the epithelium and attempted to separate the cells into five groups (normal, koilocytosis, CIN I, CIN II, CIN III). Stepwise discriminant analysis found that epithelial cell area and nuclear to cytoplasmic ratio were the two best features to distinguish between koilocytosis and CIN I. Nuclear area squared to cytoplasmic ratio and the ratio between mean lower triangle edge length and mean upper triangle edge length were found to be the best features to distinguish between CIN I, II and III. In separating CIN III from normality, these two features and epithelial area were found to be the strongest features. Unfortunately, the results were not as good as one would hope. One must bear in mind that this work was conducted on histological images of cervical specimens. Of the 30 normal images and 46 CIN III images, their system demonstrated 98.7% accuracy. This is a good result but these are visually quite different entities and not diagnostically difficult. Only 62.3% of the 142 CIN images were correctly classified. In distinguishing 76 combined images of koilocytosis and normality, the accuracy was 76.5%. They attributed their poor results to interobserver variation in the diagnosis of CIN, and the difficulties in defining distinct cutoff points in a continuous spectrum of disease. A critical deficiency in their methodology is the lack of comparison of cases with reactive hyperplasia, and immature squamous metaplasia both of which superficially can resemble CIN III.

The potential role of medical vision systems in diagnostic pathology practice

The role of medical vision systems in pathology is not to replace the pathologist, or even to modify his/her existing work practice. Instead, medical vision systems should be there to assist the pathologist, working in the background as a 'silent invigilator'. The closest analogy is to the ubiquitous yet unassuming spelling checker present in contemporary word processors. It draws attention to possible spelling errors and provides alternatives when possible.

We are familiar with the typical chain of events from when a patient presents with a suspicious mass (Figure 1). Although the diagnostic pathologist can call upon several sources of knowledge, the path to an accurate diagnosis is not always straight and there are many factors that can interfere with the diagnostic process (Figure 2). Pathologists are fallible. Fatigue and boredom are potential causes of error, especially with high volume repetitive cases as has been demonstrated with the cytological screening of cervical smears. In histopathology, there are fewer examples of repetitive work but fatigue and boredom can equally develop after a few hours of continuous examination of histological sections.

Figure 1. The flow of events from when a suspicious mass is identified by a clinician

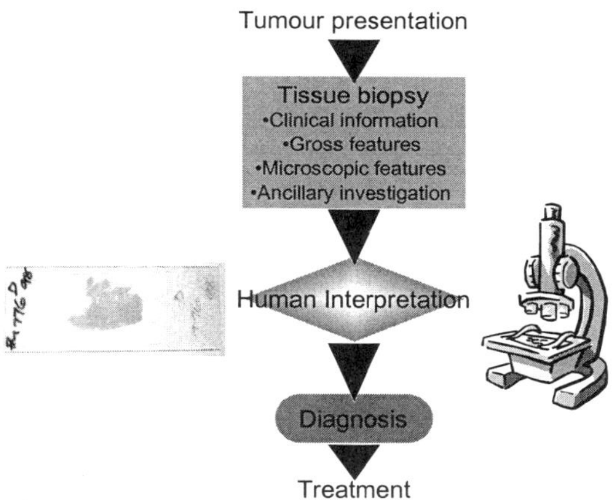

Figure 2. Possible pathways to histopathological diagnosis

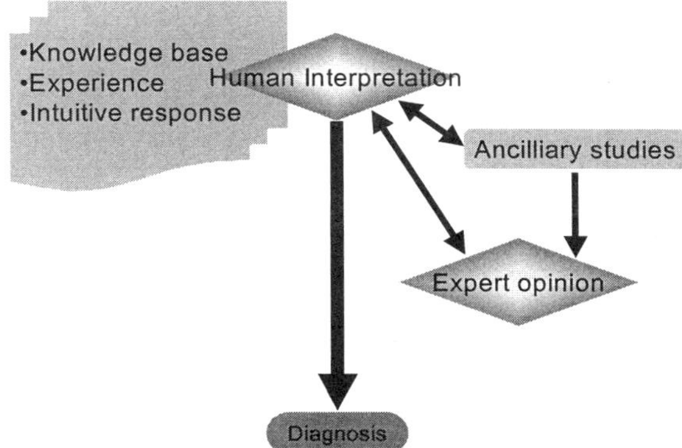

The source of error may not always originate with the pathologist. Laboratory error can result in the patient being assigned another person's specimen and therefore the wrong clinical history. With certain types of histopathology specimens such as follow-up biopsies or organ transplant, the results of past pathology reports are needed in order to interpret findings correctly or for comparison of progression of the condition.

Figure 3. Sources of error in histological interpretation

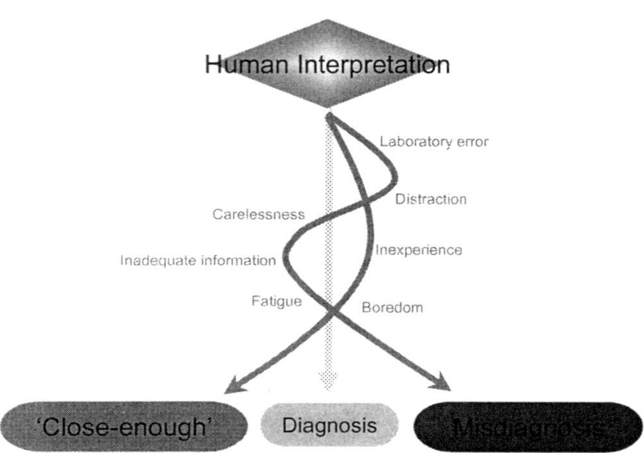

There is also potential danger in the mundane side of things. Much of a general pathologist's caseload is referred to as 'routine' work. These could best be described as cases in which the time spent on screening all the slides, administration and paperwork far exceeds the time spent reaching a diagnosis. Examples include the examination of benign melanocytic naevi, gastric and duodenal biopsies, colonic biopsies from multiple locations for non-specific diarrhoea or weight loss, bone chips for bone bank screening, bronchial biopsies for bronchitis, and endometrial curettings. The prevalence of neoplasia among all such cases is often low and the range of possible non-neoplastic diagnoses narrow. Having to deal with a monotonous stream of routine cases can dull a pathologist's sensitivity for detecting the minority with more serious pathologies. A heavy caseload will also increase the likelihood of fatigue and all the negative aspects associated with this.

Finally, limited experience increases the likelihood of error when the pathological condition is rare or when it is an unusual presentation of a common condition. A junior pathologist or one who has only worked in centres where the range of cases is restricted, will have a smaller internal visual database to complement his knowledge base than, say, one who is much more experienced and has been exposed to a wider variety of diseases and situations in many different centres.

What is also interesting is that experienced pathologists will develop strong intuitive feelings about certain diagnoses. Although they will adhere to standard practice and order relevant tests to exclude other diagnoses, this is often more to satisfy medico-legal requirements rather than to assist them in their interpretations. Is this a manifestation of higher-level image recognition skills derived through experience or is this a false confidence arising from the arrogance or complacency of familiarity? There are no studies that have investigated this properly. Indeed one of the hallmarks of 'expertise' is that it appears effortless, and that knowledge is mobilised through thought processes that are not easily explained. While experts have consummate skill, this does not always equate with an ability to introspect and articulate their thought processes.

We could speculate that there may be more diagnostic information in a histological image that the normal histopathologist is able to utilise and that with greater experience his or her recognition skills begin to operate at a more sophisticated level than he was originally taught. If this were the case then such data could be utilised by a machine vision system, provided it were correctly identified beforehand. Nonetheless, we can see there are many circumstances where errors may occur (Figure 3). Fortunately for the patient, even when errors occur, the end result is usually a diagnosis that may not be highly specific but is useable by the attending clinicians and most importantly, *does no harm* to the patient. An example is inflammatory skin disease, where the treatment is the same for a large number of conditions. In other situations, the end-result is a misdiagnosis that has clinical implications that harm the patient. An example of this is the failure to detect an abnormal cervical smear or misdiagnosing a physiological condition as a malignancy that results in disfiguring or debilitating surgery.

While a computer system is incapable of taking into consideration all the factors that may assist decision-making for a pathologist, its consistency and lack of susceptibility to extraneous influences make it a quantitative, precise and repeatable aid in the diagnostic process. Furthermore, every pathologist requires to be trained to acquire the necessary diagnostic skills through the accumulation of factual knowledge and experience. In addition to being a tool in routine clinical diagnosis, a computer database could also be utilised for the teaching of new pathologists, potentially having the capability of demonstrating a wide range of conditions and multiple variations of the same condition.

An automated recognition system or computer-aided method of diagnosis can thus act as a 'safety-net' for the working pathologist (Figure 4) we see the future role of image analysis as providing assistance to a pathologist (not as a replacement for), as also making explicit the diagnostic process and describing this process in new terms that are objective, reproducible and quantifiable.

Figure 4. By acting as a 'safety-net', enhancing the human pathologist, a computer-based diagnostic support system can potentially eliminate most common sources of error, resulting in higher diagnostic accuracy

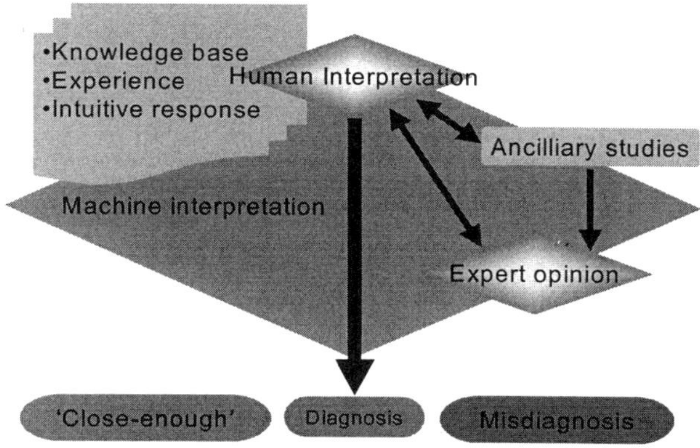

There has been much commercial promotion of automated cervical cytology screeners from companies such as Tripath Imaging (Neopath and Autocyte) and the now-defunct Papnet. In cytology, automation is not just a desire; it is a necessity in some areas where there is a shortfall of qualified cytology screeners. Automated immunostain quantification units are marketed alongside automated immunostain units. These have had a mixed response in the immunohistology community and claim to offer a degree of objectivity in the assessment of immunostain stain intensity, a necessary activity in routine diagnostic practice. Both of these technologies have managed to gain a limited acceptance in the pathology laboratory by offering functionality that assists the pathologist. At present, there is no commercially-available automated analysis/diagnostic system for breast histopathology or for that matter, for any diagnostic histopathological process.

Materials and Methods

The source material used in this project originated from United Kingdom NEQAS (National External Quality Assurance Scheme) archives, local files and 'expert' pathologist collections. In order to set a baseline standard, UK National Health Service Breast Screening Programme NEQAS and local histology slides served as the initial sample dataset. The former sample set has the benefit of consensus expert opinion, that is, the opinion of an expert panel of twenty specialist breast pathologists (members of the Breast Screening Programme Pathology committee).

Cases from contributing pathologists brought the total to 32 separate slides. These were randomised and separated into two groups. One group was used for deriving and calculating relevant features; the second group was used for system testing. The total number of digital images acquired from these samples is recorded in subsequent discussion.

Tubular carcinoma is relatively uncommon and also invariably a small lesion, usually <2cm in maximum dimension. Nonetheless, even with a single slide of average dimensions, it is possible to digitise multiple different views of the tumour at different magnifications.

Matlab (Release 11, Mathworks, Natick, Massachusetts) was used to apply the image processing algorithms. Matlab software is a versatile tool for mathematical computing and contains its own technical language for programming. It is optimised to handle multi-dimensional numerical matrices, and as this is the most common way for quantifying a digital colour image, it is well suited for image data manipulation and analysis.

The digital camera used for the majority of the images was a ProgRes 3012 (originally Kontron Electronik, now produced by Jenoptik, Germany), a progressive-scan CCD digital camera with a digital connection to the computer. Size of image capture may be set from 512 pixels x 387 pixels x 36 bit colour (0.6 megabytes) up to 4608 x 3480 x 36 bit (47 megabytes). The camera was mounted via 'C-mount' adaptor on a Leitz Laborlux 12 microscope with Fluorite-type objective lenses (4x/Numerical aperture NA 0.12, 10x/NA 0.25, 25x/NA 0.50, 40x/NA 0.70).

A variety of different techniques were used to achieve unsupervised segmentation of diagnostic features at both low and high-power levels. A detailed discussion of technique is not possible in this article.

We intuitively chose a set of features and assessed their expression in both benign and malignant training images in order to determine their relative significance. This information was then used to set the parameters within the system. Features tested included:

- Cluster area
- Number of glands in a cluster
- Gland area – range, average, standard deviation

- Total gland area: Cluster area
- Glandular maximum and minimum dimensions, eccentricity, orientation
- Mean distance from centroid of cluster (normalised)
- Proportion of glands with a single, sharply angled edge

The important processes within this system are outlined in Figure 8. We stress the multi-component nature of this system. Each component utilises information derived from previous components. The impact of any weaknesses in a single component is reduced by the fact that no one single processing step determines the final interpretation, it is the cumulative data derived from multiple stages of interpretation. This approach also permits modification and refinement of individual components or new components to be added later. The following paragraphs describe the components of the system, which essentially worked at two magnifications:

Interpretation of the low-power image

There is no formal definition for 'low-power' although many microscopists regard this as an objective magnification less than 10x ('10 times'). We define 'low-power' as being the magnification at which glandular outlines are distinct and there is sufficient field-of-view to discern overall tumour architecture. This corresponds to a 4x objective lens on most microscopes.

Much of the analysis therefore involved relative rather than absolute measures, allowing the results to be useful even if the digital imaging apparatus changes. Where absolute measurements were necessary, prior calibration was used to maintain consistency. This approach allows the system to operate independent of hardware.

The steps undertaken at low-power are as follows:

Segmentation of glandular and stromal features

Segmentation partitions an image into its constituent parts. The purpose of this phase is to accentuate the diagnostic features of the image in order to maximise the results of subsequent processes. Histopathological images are highly textured and rich with salient information. Segmentation of features is not straightforward and cannot be achieved in an automated manner using existing commercial image analysis software or applying standard image processing routines.

Much depends on effective segmentation. Initially, manual segmentation was performed and used as a baseline to compare the efficacy of different image processing segmentation methods. This was a design strategy – to firstly develop an overall architecture, develop components within this framework, demonstrate that these components produced useful data, and then automate the processes.

Division into cluster groups

The normal histology of the breast demonstrates glandular acinar structures feeding into collecting ducts. What we see under the microscope is a two-dimensional slice through these structures. It possible to recognise benign aggregates by the way the orderly architecture of glands aggregating around a central point. With malignant disease, consistent patterns are less obvious, however if we work on the premise that malignancy begins from a single point, then with smaller lesions, such as tubular carcinomas, in certain circumstances, apparent groups or clusters may be evident. What is really happening is that the tumour is growing abnormal tubules outwards from a point of origin. Although this growth is random and haphazard, in a random section through the tumour it is often still possible to discern aggregates of glands (Figure 5). However, this is not always the case as Figure 6 demonstrates. The nature of malignant glands is to infiltrate between normal structures and under these circumstances separation of malignant glands from benign clusters on a gland-by-gland basis becomes difficult. In such circumstances the image was considered as a single cluster.

Figure 5. Image demonstrating four apparent 'clusters' or glandular aggregates. The three benign (B) groups are distinct and somewhat orderly but the malignant aggregate (M) is less so.

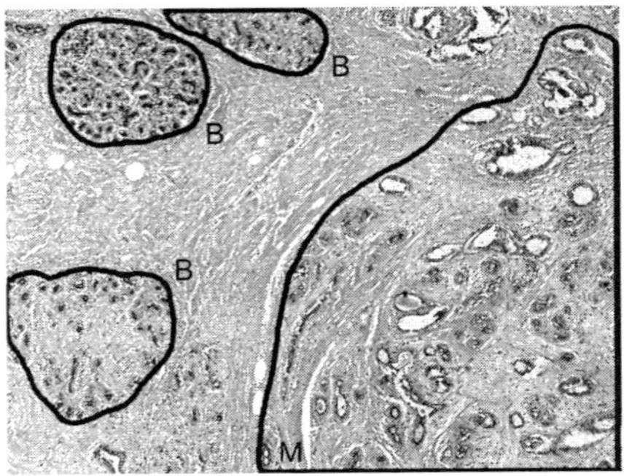

Figure 6. In contrast with Figure 5, tumour glands are diffusely distributed through this particular field of view and it is not easy to visually separate invasive from benign or in situ groups.

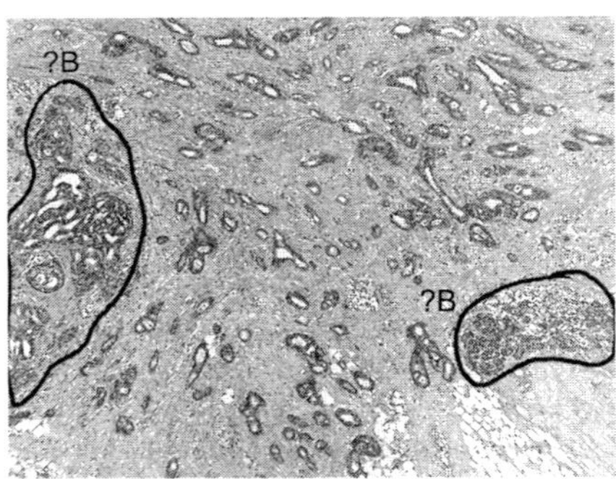

Feature selection within individual groups

Having divided the image into groups of glands, each cluster was considered separately. The histological features assessed included glandular size, shape, orientation, number, area, and density. The features that were found to assist in separating a malignant glandular cluster from a benign one were the size of the cluster, the size of individual glands, the shape of individual glands and the pattern of infiltration. Based on this data, clusters were classified as either benign or suspicious (high probability for malignancy).

Request random high-power image of suspicious cluster

A histopathologist will be able to make most diagnoses using low-power examinations; however, it is necessary to use a high-power image to confirm an initial impression or to assess prognostic factors such as mitotic activity or pleomorphism.

This system works on a similar principle. Having assessed the low-power image a request is made for randomly selected high-power image in the region determined to have a high probability of malignancy on the basis of the results from the previous step.

Image interpretation at high-power

High-power image interpretation follows a similar procedure to low-power interpretation. However, the scale is different and given that the images analysed at this stage have already been screened with low-power analysis, the incidence of malignancy is likely to be higher and suspicion must be higher. There are several features that distinguish a malignant tubular carcinoma gland from a benign gland at high-power. These include the absence of basal lamina, the angular shape of the gland, and relatively enlarged epithelial cells lining the gland which may demonstrate nuclear chromatin changes such as hyperchromasia, nuclear chromatin clumping, prominent nucleoli and increased nuclear to cytoplasmic ratio.

Segmentation of features

The high-power image will allow characterisation of gland shape with great precision than at low-power. However, what is of more value is the information about cell cytology (individual cell size, nuclear size, chromatin features, nucleoli, mitoses) that can be assessed at this higher resolution.

Detection of nucleoli

Malignant cells frequently have prominent nucleoli. It is not always present and to a certain extent, detection of nucleoli is affected by the histochemical stain, tissue section illumination under the microscope, microscope optical quality, and digital camera sensitivity.

Nucleoli detection was based upon thresholding the nuclear luminance intensities at increasing intensity levels and recognising the appearance of a round shape corresponding to a nucleolus.

Assessment of basement membrane/basal lamina

Basal lamina forms a continuous layer around benign glands but is absent around invasive malignancy (in situ disease has an intact layer). It therefore can be used as a strong feature to recognise benign glands. The detection of basal lamina is visually difficult with routine histochemical stains and immunohistochemistry has been the gold-standard. However, using image processing, basement membrane can be approximated and this derived feature is used as a strong discriminant.

The technique for approximating basement membrane was compared against immunostaining with type IV collagen and alpha-smooth muscle actin.

Results

Given word length restrictions, this article will not be able to discuss all the results thoroughly. Instead we will mention a few areas of interest:

Features found to be useful in distinguishing tubular carcinoma from benign at low power

Sixty-two benign glandular clusters and 52 malignant clusters were assessed. The significant parameters found to discriminate tubular carcinoma from benign conditions included >20% of glands with sharp-angled edge, cluster area >150,000 pixels (relative to scale used), ratio total gland area:total cluster area <0.14, >60 glands per cluster and the ratio average malignant gland area:benign gland area <0.5. The following measured or calculated features were found to be poor predictors of malignancy with unacceptably low sensitivity and specificity:

- Maximum/minimum/mean/median gland long axis lengths
- Maximum/minimum/mean/median gland short axis lengths
- Minimum/maximum/mean gland eccentricity.

(This is the eccentricity of an equivalent ellipse matching the gland outline. The eccentricity is the ratio of the distance between the foci of the ellipse and its major axis length. An ellipse whose eccentricity is 0 is actually a circle, while an ellipse whose eccentricity is 1 is a line segment).

- Maximum/minimum/mean normalised distance from each gland centroid to cluster centroid
- Comparative standard deviations of all the above parameters

Glandular orientation (cumulative, mean, standard deviation) calculated by eigen vectors or by long/short axis determination was also not found to be a useful feature. Eigen vectors calculated on stroma alone, or in combination with glands was similarly unremarkable, or rather, no discernible difference could be ascertained between benign and malignant images.

Receiver operating characteristic curves allowed the determination of the best criteria to apply and these are summarised in Table 1.

Table 1. Summary of objective distinguishing features that allow separation of tubular carcinoma from benign breast glandular aggregates

Criteria	Features associated with tubular carcinoma	Calculated likelihood ratio[*]	Area under graph (A_z)[**]
1	>20% of the glands have a sharp-angled edge	61	0.99
2	Cluster area is > 150,000 square pixels	61	0.99
3	Ratio of total gland area to total cluster area < 0.14	56	0.96
4	>60 glands per cluster	28	0.89
5	Average malignant gland area (with lumen included) : average benign gland area < 0.5	1.7	0.54

[*]Likelihood ratio is calculated from ROC curves
[**]Area under the graph also calculated from ROC curves and is a measure of how good a test is. The closer to one, the better the test.

Automated gland cluster recognition

This was achieved using a combination of Gaussian smoothing and colour quantisation and demonstrated 100% accuracy in identifying glandular aggregates within an image. In those images where glands were present in a diffuse manner without obvious clustering, a preceeding step was implemented of identifying these through nearest-neighbour and variance measurements of gland nuclei positioning [43]. This was found to be 100% effective in distinguishing images which contained diffuse tumour, and no clustering.

Accuracy of glandular segmentation using nonlinear diffusion smoothing

A total of 7973 glands were counted manually in 27 benign and 62 tubular carcinoma images. There were 643 incompletely-segmented glands (8.1%). One hundred and sixty-eight glands were missed. The majority of these glands were smaller than average size (<75 pixels area). There were also 242 instances of false segmentation, that is, segmentation of stroma features. Many of these appeared adjacent fat lobules and may have been inflammatory cells.

Feature analysis at high-power magnification

Suspicious clusters were subjected to high-power feature analysis for nuclear morphology, nucleoli detection and basement membrane assessment. Watershed thresholding achieved nuclear segmentation and progressive thresholding was used to detect nucleoli (Figure 7). Basement membrane was accentuated by colour segmentation and demonstrated 0.96 sensitivity, 0.89 specificity and 0.92 positive predictive value for distinguishing malignancy.

Figure 7. Progressive thresholding (increments of 5) to detect nucleoli. (a) is a benign nucleus. No nucleoli were detected. (b) is a malignant nucleus. A single prominent nucleolus is the first to appear and maintains a steady shape and size over several levels.

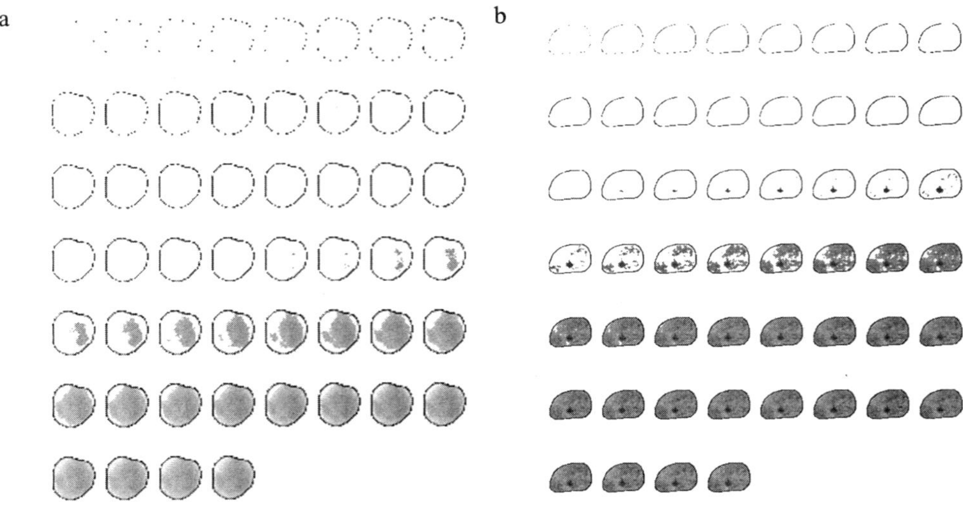

Figure 8. System overview. This outlines the important steps or components within the system framework.

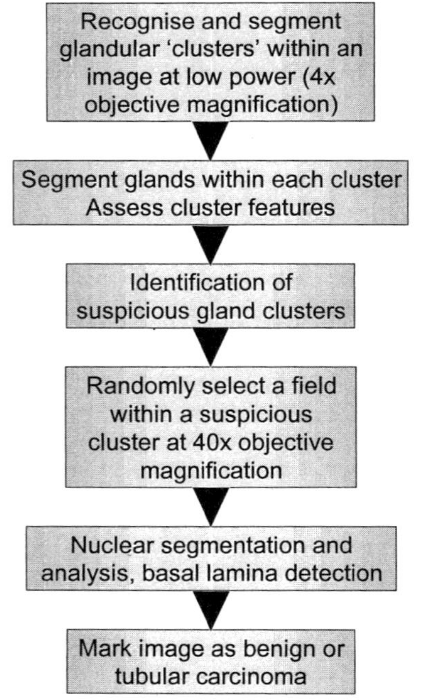

Following Laplacian filtering, benign nuclei had a mean value of 619 ±120 while the malignant set had a mean value of 732 ± 77. An ROC curve analysis of the data revealed this feature to be a feature of moderate value. From the curve, a mean value greater than 675 has a 2.75 times likelihood of belonging to a malignant category.

There was no significant difference between benign and malignant nuclei on the basis of eccentricity; however, there was a significant difference in size as determined by relative area and equivalent diameter. An area greater than 1.4 times the mean benign nuclear area is highly specific for malignancy. Equivalent diameter is often easier to measure than area. A value greater than 1.2 times that of the mean benign equivalent diameter almost certainly belongs to a malignant cell (specificity = 1).

Within the test set of 30 benign and 30 malignant nuclei, there were 16 nucleoli in total within in 14 malignant nuclei. All 16 nucleoli were detected successfully.

Overall, provided information from everyone component was utilised, the system was able to classify 135 images with 100% accuracy (49 benign, 86 tubular carcinomas). This is a small test set but the results are promising.

Conclusions

The ability of the histopathologist to assess a histological slide is sophisticated and complex and should not be over-simplified. Nonetheless, if a lesion has a set of features then these may be quantified and assessed. This work lays groundwork for further research working towards a time when histological interpretations may take place without subjective influences.

It will be some time before automated histopathology systems become widespread and reach a level where they will replace humans. Even if such systems were commercially available and sufficiently accurate, they would not be immediately accepted. Therefore, the less-threatening role for an automated diagnostic system would be as a support system, interceding only to prevent diagnostic errors.

We focussed on a single tumour as it was unfeasible within the time period to consider all tumours even within a single organ system. An alternative approach would have been to develop a system that was able to broadly classify images into benign and malignant categories. However, the value of such a system is debatable. It would potentially be able to function as a screening tool but screening a section of breast for tumour requires far less time that a cervical smear and the current demand for such a tool is low. It is possible though that automated screening of breast slides for tumour would have application in frozen section assessment of surgical margins, or detecting micrometastases in a series of axillary lymph node dissections. The idea of frozen section assessment by machine is potentially-attractive to the surgeon.

While it is possible to make some generalisations to separate malignant from benign lesions, it would demonstrate only a superficial understanding of histopathology. There are inevitably lesions that will not conform with general rules. The fact that there are entire textbooks devoted to the subject of breast disease should indicate that tumour-specific profiling is a more-comprehensive approach that will allow for adaptation as tumour classification evolves. Lesion-specific profiling would also allow a system to incorporate the spectrum of in situ breast disease. We chose to use tubular carcinoma for its distinct pattern and appearances. Many of the features will be present in other epithelial lesions.

For it to act as a support system as we had originally proposed, it must be as accurate as a pathologist but also as fast. Real-time imaging and image processing would be necessary. One area we have not discussed is the acceptability to a diagnostic pathologist. To use an artificial support may be perceived as an admission of weakness. On the other hand, it may also be viewed as good medicolegal practice. An alternative application of an automated diagnostic system is in image database cataloguing. Large collections of images are underutilised simply because the images are not indexed, a labour-intensive exercise requiring interpretive skills.

The H&E stain remains the central medium for primary interpretation, but for how much longer? In the field of radiology, a single plain x-ray film is no longer regarded as the best method of imaging but remains in use due to the infrastructure and trained staffed who have based their careers around it. Even so, radiologists are open to new imaging techniques and not adverse to questioning the way their images are derived. We believe that histopathologists should follow similar principles if the specialty is to evolve.

References

[1] Bacus JW, Belanger MG, Aggarwal RK, Trobaugh FE, Jr. Image processing for automated erythrocyte classification. J Histochem Cytochem 1976;24:195-201.

[2] Bartels PH, Bibbo M, Graham A, Paplanus S, Shoemaker RL, Thompson D. Image understanding system for histopathology. Anal Cell Pathol 1989;1:195-214.

[3] Bartels PH, Hiessl H. Expert systems in histopathology. II. Knowledge representation and rule-based systems. Anal Quant Cytol Histol 1989;11:147-53.

[4] Bartels PH, Thompson D. Expert systems in histopathology. III. Representation of knowledge as 'structured objects'. Anal Quant Cytol Histol 1989;11:367-74.

[5] Bartels PH, Thompson D, Bartels HG, Shoemaker R. Machine vision system for diagnostic histopathology. Pathol Res Pract 1989;185:635-46.

[6] Bartels PH, Thompson D, Weber JE. Expert systems in histopathology. IV. The management of uncertainty. Anal Quant Cytol Histol 1992;14:1-13.

[7] Bartels PH, Thompson D, Bibbo M, Weber JE. Bayesian belief networks in quantitative histopathology. Anal Quant Cytol Histol 1992;14:459-73.

[8] Bartels PH, Thompson D, Weber JE. Expert systems in histopathology. V. DS theory, certainty factors and possibility theory. Anal Quant Cytol Histol 1992;14:165-74.

[9] Bartels PH, Thompson D, Weber JE. Construction of the knowledge file for an image understanding system. Pathol Res Pract 1992;188:396-404.

[10] Bartels PH. Computer-generated diagnosis and image analysis. An overview. Cancer 1992;69:1636-8.

[11] Bartels PH, Thompson D, Weber JE. Diagnostic decision support by inference networks. In Vivo 1993;7:379-85.

[12] Bartels PH, Thompson D, Montironi R, Hamilton PW, Scarpelli M. Diagnostic decision support for prostate lesions. Pathol Res Pract 1995;191:945-57.

[13] Bartels PH, Thompson D, Bartels HG, Montironi R, Scarpelli M, Hamilton PW. Machine vision-based histometry of premalignant and malignant prostatic lesions. Pathol Res Pract 1995;191:935-44.

[14] Bartels PH, Thompson D, Weber JE. Diagnostic and prognostic decision support systems. Pathologica 1995;87:221-36.

[15] Bartels PH, Thompson D, Montironi R. Knowledge-based image analysis in the precursors of prostatic adenocarcinoma. Eur Urol 1996;30:234-42.

[16] Bartels PH, Thompson D, Montironi R, Mariuzzi G, Hamilton PW. Automated reasoning system in histopathologic diagnosis and prognosis of prostate cancer and its precursors. Eur Urol 1996;30:222-33.

[17] Bartels PH, Gahm T, Thompson D. Automated microscopy in diagnostic histopathology: From image processing to automated reasoning. Int J Imaging Syst Technol 1997;8:214-23.

[18] Bartels PH, Montironi R, Hamilton PW, Thompson D, Vaught L, Bartels HG. Nuclear chromatin texture in prostatic lesions. II. PIN and malignancy associated changes. Anal Quant Cytol Histol 1998;20:397-406.

[19] Bartels PH, Montironi R, Hamilton PW, Thompson D, Vaught L, Bartels HG. Nuclear chromatin texture in prostatic lesions. I. PIN and adenocarcinoma. Anal Quant Cytol Histol 1998;20:389-96.

[20] Bartels PH, da Silva VD, Montironi R, Hamilton PW, Thompson D, Vaught L, et al. Chromatin texture signatures in nuclei from prostate lesions. Anal Quant Cytol Histol 1998;20:407-16.

[21] Bartels PH, Montironi R, Thompson D, Vaught L, Hamilton PW. Statistical histometry of the basal cell/secretory cell bilayer in prostatic intraepithelial neoplasia. Anal Quant Cytol Histol 1998;20:381-8.

[22] Bartels PH, Bartels HG, Montironi R, Hamilton PW, Thompson D. Machine vision in the detection of prostate lesions in histologic sections. Anal Quant Cytol Histol 1998;20:358-64.

[23] Bartels PH, Bibbo M, Hutchinson ML, Gahm T, Grohs HK, Gwi-Mak E, et al. Computerized screening devices and performance assessment: development of a policy towards automation. International Academy of Cytology Task Force summary. Diagnostic Cytology Towards the 21st Century: An International Expert Conference and Tutorial. Acta Cytol 1998;42:59-68.

[24] Thompson D, Bartels PH, Bartels HG, Montironi R. Knowledge-guided histometry of the basal cell layer in prostatic intraepithelial neoplasia. Anal Quant Cytol Histol 1996;18:177-84.

[25] Thompson D, Bartels PH, Bartels HG, Hamilton PW, Sloan JM. Knowledge-guided segmentation of colorectal histopathologic imagery. Anal Quant Cytol Histol 1993;15:236-46.

[26] Bibbo M, Xiao J, Christen R, Fitzpatrick B, Galera-Davidson H, Bartels PH, et al. Use of computer graphic filters for the nuclear grading of hematoxylin and eosin-stained specimens from prostatic lesions. Anal Quant Cytol Histol 1994;16:183-8.

[27] Christen R, Xiao J, Minimo C, Gibbons G, Fitzpatrick BT, Galera-Davidson H, et al. Chromatin texture features in hematoxylin and eosin-stained prostate tissue. Anal Quant Cytol Histol 1993;15:383-8.

[28] Mairinger T, Mikuz G, Gschwendtner A. Nuclear chromatin texture analysis of nonmalignant tissue can detect adjacent prostatic adenocarcinoma. Prostate 1999;41:12-9.

[29] Scarpelli M, Montironi R, Mazzucchelli R, Thompson D, Bartels PH. Distinguishing cortical adrenal gland adenomas from carcinomas by their quantitative nuclear features. Anal Quant Cytol Histol 1999;21:131-8.

[30] Scarpelli M, Montironi R, Thompson D, Bartels PH. Computer-assisted analysis of medulloblastoma. A cytologic study. Anal Quant Cytol Histol 1997;19:387-92.

[31] Scarpelli M, Montironi R, Thompson D, Bartels PH. Computer-assisted discrimination of glioblastomas. Anal Quant Cytol Histol 1997;19:369-75.

[32] Esgiar AN, Naguib RN, Sharif BS, Bennett MK, Murray A. Microscopic image analysis for quantitative measurement and feature identification of normal and cancerous colonic mucosa. IEEE Trans Inf Technol Biomed 1998;2:197-203.

[33] Dawson AE, Austin RE, Jr., Weinberg DS. Nuclear grading of breast carcinoma by image analysis. Classification by multivariate and neural network analysis. Am J Clin Pathol 1991;95:S29-37.

[34] Dawson AE, Cibas ES, Bacus JW, Weinberg DS. Chromatin texture measurement by Markovian analysis. Analyt Quant Ctyol Histol 1993;15:227-35.

[35] Albert R, Muller JG, Kristen P, Harms H. Objective nuclear grading for node-negative breast cancer patients: comparison of quasi-3D and 2D image-analysis based on light microscopic images. Lab Invest 1998;78:247-59.

[36] Weyn B, van de Wouwer G, van Daele A, Scheunders P, van Dyck D, van Marck E, et al. Automated breast tumor diagnosis and grading based on wavelet chromatin texture description. Cytometry 1998; 33:32-40.

[37] Van De Wouwer G, Weyn B, Scheunders P, Jacob W, Van Marck E, Van Dyck D. Wavelets as chromatin texture descriptors for the automated identification of neoplastic nuclei. J Microsc 2000;197:25-35.

[38] Montironi R, Whimster WF, Collan Y, Hamilton PW, Thompson D, Bartels PH. How to develop and use a Bayesian Belief Network. J Clin Pathol 1996;49:194-201.

[39] Montironi R, Bartels PH, Hamilton PW, Thompson D. Atypical adenomatous hyperplasia (adenosis) of the prostate: development of a Bayesian belief network for its distinction from well-differentiated adenocarcinoma. Hum Pathol 1996;27:396-407.

[40] Hamilton PW, Montironi R, Abmayr W, Bibbo M, Anderson N, Thompson D, et al. Clinical applications of Bayesian belief networks in pathology. Pathologica 1995;87:237-45.

[41] Hamilton PW, Anderson NH, Diamond J, Bartels PH, Gregg JB, Thompson D, et al. An interactive decision support system for breast fine needle aspiration cytology. Anal Quant Cytol Histol 1996;18:185-90.

[42] Keenan SJ, Diamond J, Glenn McCluggage W, Bharucha H, Thompson D, Bartels PH, et al. An automated machine vision system for the histological grading of cervical intraepithelial neoplasia (CIN). J Pathol 2000;192:351-62.

[43] Schwarz H, Exner H. The characterization of the arrangement of feature centroids in planes and volumes. J Microsc 1983;129:155.

Acknowledgements

Histological materials were obtained from the archives of the UK Breast National External Quality Assurance Scheme. The following pathologists also provided additional histological materials:
- Professor Anthony Leong (Newcastle, New South Wales, Australia)
- Dr Ian Ellis (Nottingham, UK)
- Dr Tom Anderson (Edinburgh, UK)

Professor JM Brady (Oxford University Engineering Sciences) provided invaluable advice and this work would not have been possible without his guidance.

Address for Correspondence

Professor James O'D McGee
University of Oxford
Nuffield Department of Medicine
John Radcliffe Hospital
Oxford OX3 9DU, United Kingdom
phone: +44 1865 220549
fax: +44 1865 222901
e.mail: James.McGee@ndm.ox.ac.uk

Integration of Health Telematics into Medical Practice
M. Nerlich and U. Schaechinger (Eds.)
IOS Press, 2003

Data Analysis Now and Then: Significant Changes in Approaches and Results

MARKUS T. J. MOHR[1], HEINZ REDL[2]

[1] *BioMedical Data Processing Group (BMDPG), Regensburg (Director: Dr. M. T. J. Mohr), Spiegelgasse 1, 93047 Regensburg, Germany*
[2] *Ludwig-Boltzmann Institute for Experimental and Clinical Traumatology, (Heads: Prof. Dr. H. Redl, Dr. A. Kroepfl), Donaueschingenstrasse 13, 1200 Vienna, Austria*

Abstract. Modern data analysis is one of the many prerequisites for telemedical applications. Classical statistical methods alone are no longer sufficient to fulfill the various demands of modern analytical procedures. Cluster and association analysis among others have filled this gap and are capable of producing more adequate and better suitable results as well as to provide information not detectable in the past.

Introduction

Data analysis techniques about 10 years ago were characterized by a combination of classical statistical methods and applications from "Artificial Intelligence" (AI) for improvement of results. However, for many attempts to predict the outcome of severe clinical conditions, such as sepsis and similar consuming diseases, results often were poor and inferior to human expert assessment (intuition) alone.

Using more recent forms of data analysis and evaluation, such as Neuronal Networks (NN), Fuzzy Logic (FL), Fuzzy Neuro Networks (FNN), Genetic Algorithms (GA), or Associative Cluster Analysis (ACA), better results are obtainable.

But modern methodologies often are more complex to establish, require more computational resources, and are by far more expensive.

Materials and Methods

In a data record set of 50 polytraumatized patients, 30 of whom developed trauma-associated sepsis, without further preselection the target variable "mortality in dependence of the serum activity levels of elastase" was examined. Blood serum samples were drawn twice a day (in the mean). The evaluation of data was performed "with onboard means" (i. e. the commonly accepted labchem upper range value of 255 µg/l) in comparison to trend analysis, to a an expert system (ES) with refined mathematical methods and two modern associative analysis systems (AAS), the latter based on modified NN second to KOHONEN [1,2].

The goal was on the one hand to find a

1. *correlation and / or association of mortality*
2. *directly to the measured*
3. *serum activity levels of elastase*

and on the other hand to *predict mortality from day X of measurement on* (so-called end-points).

For the *ES*, we chose *VP-EXPERT v2.2* (1988). Being Prolog-based, it permitted the integration of external methodologies (using C as coding language). On the basis of simple system requirements (80386, DOS, 16 MB RAM, 1 MB harddisk, 1 floppy disk drive), we found it easy to learn, well documented (english), relatively cheap (250 Euro) and found a simple form of licensing without complex marketing structures behind. One of the main advantages of this system was its extremely fast computation capability.

For the *AAS*, we chose two software solutions: CAT-suite 0.95 (2000) (beta version for testing) and Data-Engine 3.1 (2000). The system requirements were far more demanding than those of the ES (80586, 64 MB RAM, Windows NT, 100 MB hard disk, CD-ROM drive). Both systems were not easy to learn, "rethinking" away from human intuition was required. The documentation (English) was excellent, but both systems were expensive (1.250 to 5.000 Euro) and were subject to a complex form of licensing.

Both systems, the *ES* and the *AAS*, were "top-of-the-art" in their respective time period (1988 vs. 2000).

The methodological functionality of the *ES* had to be constructed by integrating xternal C algorithms for the BAYES theorem [3] (BT), so-called "Certainty Factors" (CF) and a special form of Likelihood Ratio (LR) as well as Densities of Probability [4,5] (DP). The basic mathematical relations are depicted in figure 1.

Figure 1. Mathematical rationales

BAYES theorem:

$$P(D_i \mid e) = P(D_i) \times P(e \mid D_i) \ / \ \Sigma\, P(D_i) \times P(e \mid D_i)$$

$P(D_i)$ = a priori probability of an event D_i
$P(D_i \mid e)$ = probability of an event D_i under the premise of an evidence e
$P(e \mid D_i)$ = probability of an evidence e under the premise of an event D_i

Certainty Factor:

$$CF[h,e] = MB[h,e] - MD[h,e]$$

$CF[h,e]$ = certainty function on behalf of hypothesis h based on evidence e
$MB[h,e]$ = "measure of increased belief" in hypothesis h based on evidence e
$MD[h,e]$ = "measure of increased disbelief" in hypothesis h based on evidence e

Likelihood Ratio and Densities of Probability:

$$LR(x_0) = pr(x_0 \mid D) \ / \ pr(x_0 \mid {-}D)^2$$

$LR(x_0)$ = likelihood ratio of x
$(x_0 \mid D)$ = density function of x among ill persons at x_0
$(x_0 \mid {-}D)$ = density function of x among not ill persons at x_0
$pr(x_0 \mid D)$ = probability of the density function $(x_0 \mid D)$
$pr(x_0 \mid {-}D)$ = probability of the density function $(x0 \mid {-}D)$

In the *AAS*, first of all, a normative transformation of data had to be carried out. Next, data preparation implied the handling of raw data, of "empty" and "missing values", and the integration of human expert knowledge. Having defined the target variable "mortality vs. serum activity levels of elastase", the NN was trained against it, and by means of cluster building prototyping was achieved. Of all those data, associative analysis was performed, and further processing second to changeable (0 to 1) "measures of relevance" was carried out, consecutively. Thus, under the premise of results obtained (not all settings deliver usable results), model building as well as classifications (both part of "system learning") were permitted.

The special predicate of both *AAS* was their ability to integrate intuitive human expert knowledge in useable, i. e. computable form. Thus, a significant expansion of the *AAS* systems together with an experience-based pre-processing of the data record has been achieved.

Results

The *ES* showed a significant superiority over the simple analysis of labchem value findings and over a simple form of trend analysis. However, the isolated consideration of labchem upper limits was worthless. The observation of mean values, furthermore, showed a clear trend:

Serum activity levels of elastase ~ mortality found

This excluded, on the other hand, a prediction of the individual patient outcome.

In the very first run of the *ES*, BAYES theorem with and without LR alone did not show any significant differences of results: patients with serum activity levels of elastase higher than the labchem upper limit of 255 µg/l did not necessarily develop complications leading to mortality.

Only by adding LR and CF, it was possible to obtain a global prediction of elastase-associated mortality amounting to *39 % from day 4 on*, optimizable to *64 % by day 7 on* by adding DP. Thereafter, no further improvement of the results was achievable.

It was not surprising that those patients who developed complications leading to mortality had significantly higher mean values of serum activity levels of elastase observed than those without complications with no mortality.

The *AAS*, on the contrary, showed a strong association between the absolute concentration values of the serum activity levels of elastase and the observed mortality immediately after NN training. The clustered strength of this association had its peak (96 %) on day 5, day 7, and day 8, respectively, thus implying an *associative pattern*.

This pattern permitted a global prediction of elastase-associated mortality amounting to *96 % from day 2 on* (retrospectively) and led to a prototype model building and classification for this respective data record.

Enhanced with further data record sets from another 25 patients, the same findings were observed, thus allowing definitive model building, classification, and systematic learning of the system ("self-optimization through self-learning").

Discussion

Due to the fact, that with the *ES* there was no significant optimization of results to the BAYES theorem by adding either LR per se or the LR together with CF, Albert [6] proposed a change of concept for these situations: Use of LR on the basis of observing the mean values and computing of variance, use of prognostic intervals, and use of LR with result-borne weighting as precursor for the application of NN (then only rudimentary).

Since the examination of the proposed data record had taken place in 1990 and since the data record then amount only to 50 patients altogether, 30 of whom were suitable for evaluation, the realization of Albert's postulations did not change the definitive results.

This is most likely due to a too small overall case number (30) and too few measurement values (twice a day).

Therefore, the chance to predict mortality in this setting, amounted to 39 % after day 4, and to 64 % after day 7 of measurement. No further improvement of results was possible.

On the side of the *AAS*, of course no mathematical correlation in the sense of classical statistics was observed, therefore the results must not be understood as a classical proof in the strict sense. This makes another "rethinking" process necessary, in that proofs for data associations nowadays no longer imply strict correlations, but "merely" contain a set of associations or cohesions with their respective strengths.

Thus, both *AAS* systems were able to identify an association between the mortality of patients and their respective serum activity of elastase, and the strength of this association amounted to a maximum of 96 % after day 2 of measurements. This means that there is sufficient information and evidence from observing the serum activity levels of elastase which can be associated to the mortality of patients in a predictive strength of 96 % from day 2 of measurements on.

With this result, prototype model building and classification is possible. Using further data records from the another unselected population of polytraumatized patients with trauma-associated sepsis, both the strength of the built model and the classification can be enhanced, and the formulation of questions to the data record(s) can be refined, retro- and especially prospectively.

Conclusion

About 10 years ago, data analysis was mostly made up of seeking a statistically provable context (falsification or verification of hypotheses).

Typically based on theorems such as BAYES theorem, apparently "strange" results or uncertainties concerning these results had to be overcome by either modifying the data record (e. g. reduction of variables, enhancing the case numbers) or by using additional methodologies, such as CF, LR, or the like.

The quality of result only seldom surmounted more than 85 % predictability. Human experts, on the contrary, mostly showed comparable results in the range of 75 to 85 % predictability.

Nowadays, more detailed and thorough analyses of data records are possible by the use of NN, FL, NFL, GA, and others or combinations of these. More recent techniques such as "self-organizing maps" (SOM) even enhance the quality of result. Among others, especially associative analyses lead to predictabilities in the range of 85 to 95% even during the "first pass" of examination (i. e. without refining evaluation parameters).

But the improvement of techniques, methodologies, and procedures often involves a far more complex approach to data records nowadays than 10 years ago.

References

[1] Kohonen T: Self-Organization and Associative Memory. 3rd edition. Springer, Berlin 1989.

[2] Kohonen T: Self-Organizing Maps. Springer, Berlin 1995.

[3] Buchanan B, Shortliffe E: Rule Based Expert Systems. Stanford University Press, 1984.

[4] Radack K, et al: The likelihood ratio. An improved measure for reporting and evaluating diagnostic test results. Arch Path Lab Medicine 110 (1986), 689 - 693.

[5] Reibenegger G, et al: Generalized likelihood ratio concept and logistic regression analysis for multiple diagnostic categories. Clin Chem 35 / 6 (1989), 990 - 994.

[6] Albert A: Multivariate Interpretation of Clinical Laboratory Data. Elsevier, New York 1987.

Address for correspondence

Markus T. J. Mohr, MD
BioMedical Data Processing Group (BMDPG)
Spiegelgasse 1
D - 93047 Regensburg, Germany
phone: +49 941 5047723
fax: +49 941 5047724
email: markus.mohr@mazimoi.de

Software Agents in Surgery:
An Update

MARKUS T. J. MOHR

BioMedical Data Processing Group (BMDPG), Regensburg (Director: Dr. M. T. J. Mohr),
Spiegelgasse 1, 93047 Regensburg, Germany

Abstract. Intelligent and, thus, autonomously reacting software programs are capable of handling a lot of different tasks as has been realized in economics and network administration. The same so-called software agents can be used for a variety of organizational tasks in medicine. Some software agents already manage an individual patient's health care record from documentation to ambulant or stationary admission, surgical planning, and many other tasks which currently consume more than half of a physician's daily working time. Hence, not only a large potential of time, but also of economical savings result to the physicians' new disposition.

Introduction

Using Software Agents (SA), all kinds of information transfer in medicine can be facilitated considerably. Not only an effective resource management, but also case and disease management, document management, surgical planning, patient transport, pre- and post-hospital patient handling, and many other tasks are thus realizable easily.

Up to now, medical SA applications have been restricted to just a few programs for special tasks. By using medical SA in a more general fashion, much of the hardship arising from a variety of administrative demands in hospitals effectively can be bundled into autonomously acting software interactions.

History and Precursors

The idea of computer systems and software as "human companions" were the first incentives to construct artificial entities helping mankind with complex tasks (cf. StarTrek). Realized examples and ideal precursors to SA are *automatons, androids, humanoids, robots,* and *cyborgs.*

Many of the original ideas stem from the phantasy world of novels and TV series.

Modern Definition

Agents in technical terminology are machines, computers, or software pro- grams which carry out man-made orders or directives to accomplish defined tasks. Doing this, they make use of endogenously applied autonomous intelligence, react to environmental changes, adapt to the experiences gained during activity and interact dynamically in a form of social embeddedness.

The user of SA defines goals, which the SA attempts to fulfill rationally. To accomplish this, he often uses the interactive cooperation of several SA (*multi SA systems*). McCarthy [1] and Selfridge [2] coined the description of SA as "…. a 'soft robot' living and doing its business within the computer's world".

Properties

Typically, SA show the following characteristics:

- *Intelligence* ("computational system")
- *Longevity, Continuity*
- *Sensors* and *Effectors* for environmental interaction
- Capability of *deciding autonomously and rationally*
- *Adaptivity* and *Flexibility*
- *Character*: "Personality" and "Emotionality"
- *Non-invasiveness*
- *Respecting borders* (e. g. "robots.txt")

4 attributes characterize differences to other software (*RAAS definition*):

- *Reactivity*: Capability of selectively perceiving and consecutively acting rationally
- *Autonomy*: Ability to endogenously act rationally (Proactivity)
- *Adaptivity*: Ability to learn from experiences, gain of *Intuition*
- *Sociability*: Task-specific coexistence with other SA in order to reach one common goal or several different goals

Practical Application in Medicine

SA effectively can be used to deal with following tasks:

- Pre-hospital organization and admission
- In-hospital resource management
- Data transfer (diagnosis, administrative data) to health insurances
- Case and disease management
- Proposal of further examinations and therapeutical options
- Surgical schedule planning
- Post-hospital delivery of medical care
- Providing all kinds of electronic information (pharmaceutical, research, etc.)
- Document management, description of the entire patient inhouse workflow per case
- Acute help on behalf of "missing experts"

These tasks can, of course, be dealt with also in a medical practice, so that SA ideally represent applications for an effective *Patient-to-Physician (P2D) contact* (Figure 1).

Figure. 1 Interconnection of SA into a medical handling environment

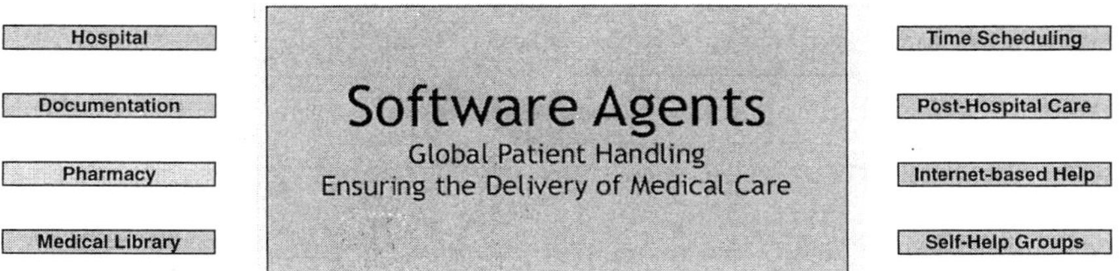

Examples

MEDICUS [2]

Medical resource and workflow planning system for operative surgery to the heart together with all necessary pre- and postoperative treatments, thus observing vital constraints. The system enables manual interaction for justifications. Special consideration for emergencies is integrated.

ChariTime [3]

Agent-oriented software system for the inhospital planning of patient time schedules (from cardiology to other disciplines), thereby planning patient examinations, optimizing workflow time and ways, effectively utilizing of existing resources and giving emergencies priority-dependent special considerations. It is equipped with an intuitive graphical user interface.

SoAS 2.5 [4]

Based on PHP, Perl, JavaScript, and C++, this SA depicts a modern Intra- and Internet-capable form of software. Its workflow comprises all of the above-mentioned tasks plus scheduled patient discharge and automatic interaction with post-hospital care taking institutions.

ABCS [5]

This agent-based computer simulation was designed to synthesize the information acquired from the linear analysis of basic science into a model that preserves the complexity of the inflammatory system. Thus, by executing several of these simulations, a more thorough understanding of sirs can evolve.

MARVIN [6]

MARVIN (Multi-Agent Retrieval Vagabond on Information Network) and is associated medical search engine MedHunt are a solution for people, who only understand a few languages, to access multilingual information throughout the world-wide web.

PatientAdvocate [7]

This system is designed to support patient's management of their own health-related behaviour on a day-to-day basis at home. Clinical treatment protocols are represented in an intention-based time-oriented representation language.

References

[1]   Computer Software. Scientific American 251 (3), 1984: 53 - 59
[2]   MEDICUS. Ein medizinisches Ressourcenplanungssystem. KI - Künstliche Intelligenz 3 (1998), 56 - 60
[3]   Proceedings of the Workshop "Agententechnologie" on the KI '99. TZI-Bericht 6/1999, 99 - 104
[4]   Informations on SoAS 2.5 can be found under: http://www.medwebdev.com
[5]   An G: Agent-based computer simulation and sirs: building a bridge between basic science and clinical trials. Shock 16 (4) 2001, 266 - 273
[6]   Baujard O, Baujard V, Aural S, Boyer S, Appel RD: MARVIN, multi-agent softbot to retrieve multilingual medical information on the Web. Med Inform 23 (3) 1998, 187 - 191
[7]   Miksch S, Cheng K, Hayes-Roth B: The patient advocate: a cooperative agent to support patient-centered needs and demands. Proc AMIA Annu Fal Symp 1996, 244 - 248

Address for correspondence

Markus T. J. Mohr, MD
BioMedical Data Processing Group (BMDPG)
Spiegelgasse 1
D - 93047 Regensburg, Germany
phone: +49 941 5047723
fax: +49 941 5047724
email: markus.mohr@mazimoi.de

Technologies for Haptic Systems in Telemedicine

GARETH J. MONKMAN[1], HOLGER BOESE[2], HELMUT ERMERT[3],
DAGMAR KLEIN[4], HERBERT FREIMUTH[4], MICHAEL BAUMANN[2],
STEFAN EGERSDOERFER[1], OTTO T. BRUHNS[3],
ALEXANDER MEIER[1], KASHIF RAJA[1]

[1]*Fachhochschule Regensburg - University of Applied Sciences, Fachbereich
Elektrotechnik, Prüfeninger Strasse 58, 93049 Regensburg, Germany*
[2]*Fraunhofer-Institut für Silicatforschung, Neunerplatz 2, 97082 Würzburg, Germany*
[3]*Ruhr-Universität Bochum, Institut fuer Hochfrequenztechnik, 44780 Bochum, Germany*
[4]*Institut für Mikrotechnik Mainz, Carl-Zeiss-Strasse 18-20, 55129 Mainz, Germany*

Abstract. The ability to image the elastic properties of tissue is potentially useful in a variety of applications. The field of elastic imaging has grown in response to the potential use of such information in medical diagnosis. Real time ultrasound elastography represents a recent development in determining strain and elasticity distributions. Nevertheless, commonly used imaging techniques rely on the interpretation of two dimensional visual data displayed on a video screen. In reality however, physicians often prefer tactile exploration making the simultaneous portrayal of both video and haptic information most desirable.

Since the 1970's many alphanumeric to tactile data conversion methods have been investigated, mainly with the ultimate aim of assisting the blind. More recently, interest has been directed toward the display of pictures on haptically explorable surfaces - Tactile imaging. Such a system would allow surgeons to examine hard sectors contained within soft tissue, and thereby assist in operations held remotely. The expansion of ultrasound elastography to 3D formats would mean the ability to haptically explore regions of the body normally inaccessible to human hands. For three-dimensional imaging the acquisition of sequential tomographic slices using Elastography, combined with image segmentation, enables the reconstruction, quantification and visualisation of tumour volumes.

In a collaborative project between four research institutes, the aim is to produce a prototype three dimensional tactile displays comprising electrically switchable micromachined cells, whose mechanical moduli are governed by phase changes experienced by electrorheological and/or magnetorheological fluids. This will be integrated with a sensory ultrasonic elastography in order to present the human fingers with controllable surfaces capable of emulating biological tissue, muscle and bone.

Introduction

Real Time Elastography. Palpation is a standard screening procedure for the detection of breast, thyroid, prostate, and liver abnormalities. The pathological state of soft tissues is often correlated with changes in stiffness, which yields a qualitative estimation of the tissues Young's modulus. However, palpation is not very accurate because of its poor sensitivity with respect to small and deeply located lesions in addition to its limited accuracy in terms of the morphological localisation of lesions. Conventional diagnostic imaging (X-ray, ultrasound, magnetic resonance imaging) are not able to visualise the mechanical tissue properties directly. Consequently, a new elastographic visualisation method based on ultrasound or magnetic resonance imaging techniques (MRI) is of growing interest. In addition to tumours situated within soft tissue, elastography is also able to detect calcifications in blood vessels; for example in the coronary arteries. The advantages of ultrasound elastography over MRI elastography is its ease of applicability and its real time capability. Real time ultrasound elastography based on high efficiency signal processing approaches [1] has recently been developed. Ultrasonic imaging is performed during compression of the medium by an external force in order to determine the strain distribution, as shown in Figure 1. Here it can be clearly seen that a rigid body in an agar-phantom is not invisible in the traditional ultrasound image. However, it can be clearly seen in the strain image to the right. In medicine for example, elastography in combination with a tactile display can assist a physician in localising tumours that are known to be stiffer than the surrounding tissue. Real time elastographic data is available from the ultrasound system in digitised RF-Data format which allows easy conversion to formats compatible with other programming systems.

Figure 1. Traditional ultrasound and strain images of a rigid body in an agar-phantom

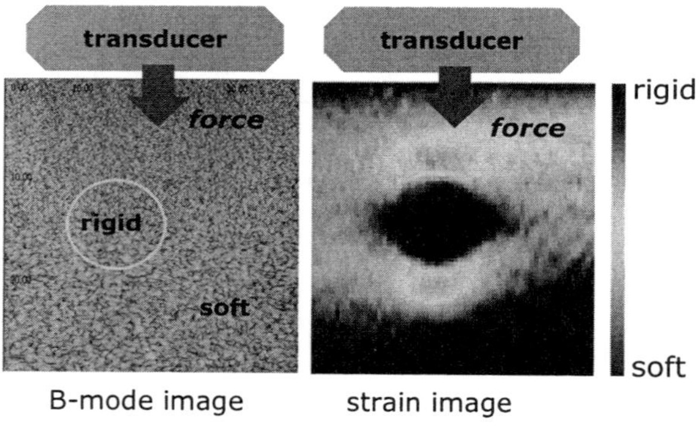

The reprojection of 2D-slices into a volume data set requires a position sensing device, which may be electromagnetic, acoustic or optical. After acquiring a series of sequential tomographic 2D-elastograms, the volume is created by placing each image at the correct location in the volume as shown in figure 2. The position data acquired with each 2D-elastogram determines the exact location of the image. Using the three dimensional volume data in building an equivalent virtual object displayed on the actively controllable 3D surface is the aim of the tactile displays.

Real time ultrasound elastography is capable of detecting prostate carcinoma with a high level of accuracy [2]. As a result the system can be used to supplement the existing methods of prostate diagnostics so as to improve the early detection of prostate cancer and allow a more reliable diagnosis. The planning of biopsies can be improved, unnecessary biopsies can be avoided and biopsies can be more reliably performed. Taken to its ultimate conclusion this will allow surgeons to obtain the impression of moving their hands through the human body in real time.

Figure 2. Reconstruction of a three-dimensional image through segmentation

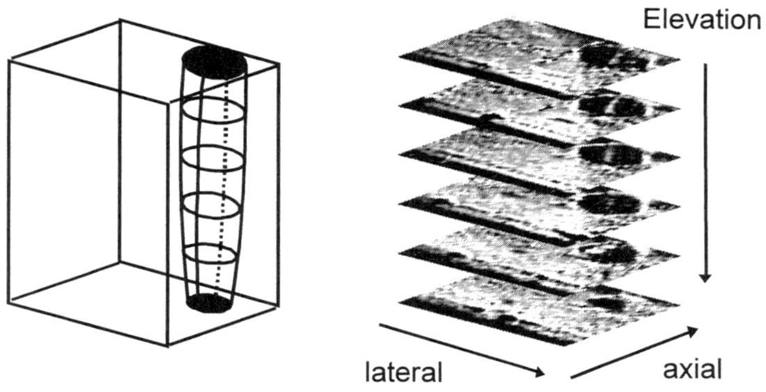

Haptic Displays

Compared to other parts of the human body, the fingertips are particularly well endowed with nerve endings. Consequently, any form of tactile display must deliver a spatial resolution of between 2 and 6 mm, depending on the vibration frequency where relevant [3]. For a haptically explorable surface a minimum of 4 by 4 elements is required and a preferred matrix size would be in the region of 16 by 16 or 32 by 32 elements. This latter would require a total of 1024 controllable elements.

Table 1. Actuators previously used in tactile displays

Physical actuation method	Array size	Typical force	Horizontal resolution	Vertical stroke	Band-width	Power/ Element
Pneumatic air jet	7 x 7	-	ca. 6.5mm	-	2 Hz	ca. 1 W
Pneumatic/hydraulic cylinder	4 x 4	2 N	4 mm	10 mm	10 Hz	0.3 W
Electromagnetic vibrator	20 x 20	0.5 N	12 mm	10 mm	100 Hz	1 W
Piezoelectric vibrator	24 x 6	0.35 N	ca. 1.5 mm	5 mm	300 Hz	0.00001 W
Thermal shape memory	8 x 8	2.5 N	2 mm	2.5 mm	<0.3 Hz	0.5 W
Pulsed electrostimulation	20 x 20	-	5 mm	-	400 Hz	0.01 W
Electrorheological Fluid	24 x 24	1 N	2.4 mm	2 mm	>20 Hz	0.02 W

To enable data to be displayed in a haptically explorable form two dimensions of horizontal spatial resolution and one dimension of controllable vertical movement are necessary. This can be achieved by means of a matrix of elements which provide a stimulus in the form of vibration or whose physical resistance to movement in the vertical plane is proportional to the elasticity of the object being portrayed. Table 1 shows actuation methods which have hitherto been investigated for the realisation of tactile display arrays.

The dimensions of the elements and arrays listed in table 1 are the actual parameters for built and tested systems - not potential maximum (or minimum) values, which may be much larger (or smaller) in other designs.

In the case of vibratory systems research suggests that the human fingers have an optimal sensitivity to vibration frequencies of around 250 Hz [4]. For movable systems, capable of portraying elasticity, several millimetres of vertical movement are required, though for simple binary displays as little as 2 mm may suffice [5].

Pneumatic

Until recently most commercially available pneumatic cylinders were far too large to provide the necessary horizontal resolution and air jets were one solution despite their very limited bandwidth [6]. Now cylinders with 2.5 mm diameter bore are commercially available [7] yielding resolutions approaching the desired 3 mm. Figure 3 shows a recently built 4 by 4 matrix employing pneumatic actuators.

Figure 3. 16 Element pneumatic/hydraulic tactile matrix.

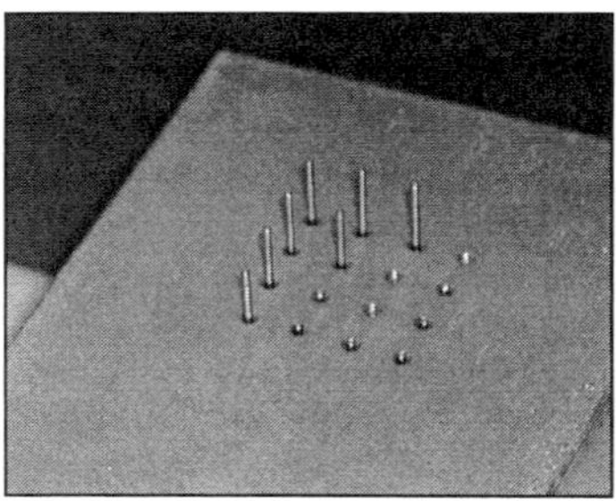
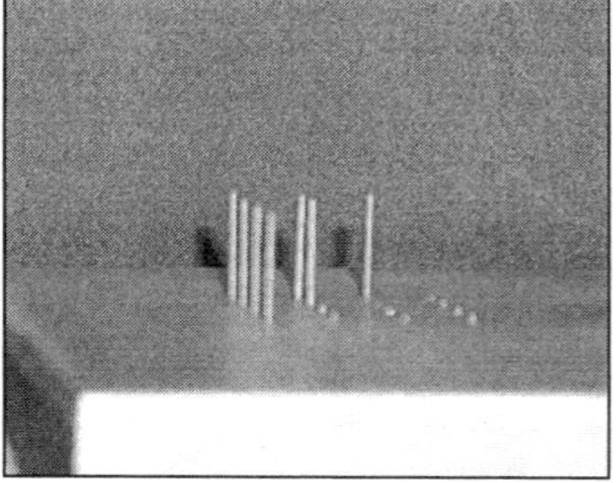

The force produced by such a cylinder can easily be calculated from expression {1} where σ is the available pneumatic pressure [N/m^2], A is the internal cylinder area, η the efficiency and F_S [N] the spring return force counteracting the applied pneumatic force.

Force, $F = \sigma\, A\, \eta - F_S$ {1}

Given a 6 bar compressed air supply a force of about 2 Newton can be expected from such a small actuator. Unfortunately air is compressible which makes it difficult to control the stroke thus limiting the vertical resolution and the reliability of hardness emulation.

A 1 cm movement in 0.1 seconds (10 Hz) from a pneumatic cylinder with an internal area of 5 mm^2 requires a volumetric air flow rate of 500 mm^3/s. For a 6 bar pressure this gives a power consumption of 300 mW per element. One thousand elements then require 300 Watts.

Hydraulic

Hydraulic actuators can be used in a similar manner, except that the incompressibility of Newtonian fluids offers some distinct advantages in that control can be exercised in the vertical plane. In fact the matrix depicted in figure 3 can just as easily be driven hydraulically as pneumatically.

Again expression {1} can be used but now the energy required is dependent on the stroke S [m] in {2} which forms part of the famous Bernoulli equation:

$$\text{Energy } e = F\,S = \sigma\,V \qquad \{2\}$$

Now in a hydraulic system the fluid must be continuously pumped. The volumetric flowrate Q [m^3 s^{-1}] and power P [W] which the pump must provide can be calculated from {3}:

$$\text{Power } P = Q\,\sigma \qquad \{3\}$$

Given a movement of 1 cm in 0.1 seconds, such an actuator will require a power of approximately 0.3 Watts and one thousand elements would again require a total pump power of 300 Watts.

Unfortunately both pneumatic and hydraulic systems suffer from one major disadvantage. They both require control valves which tend to be larger and bulkier than the actuators themselves. This inevitably results in a control unit many time larger than the display itself with additional power consumption where electromagnetically driven pneumatic or hydraulic valves are used.

Electromagnetic

Electromagnetic solenoids are also a possible solution though large strokes and/or large forces require rather bulky coils which have hitherto limited potential resolution [8]. More recently, micro sized inductors have led to the development of extremely small electromagnetic devices including micro-motors [9] but these either demand excessive power and/or tend to be relatively expensive.

There is very little on the market in the way of solenoids with diameters less than 8 mm. Furthermore, even the smallest solenoid capable of a 1 cm stroke consumes about 1 Watt of power in the on-state. A thousand elements simultaneously energised would require 1 kW!

Electrostatic

Recent developments in high dielectric constant elastomers has awakened interest in electrostatic actuators based on capacitor sandwiches. Arrays have been proposed, though it is not clear whether any working models are available. Based on available data and simple calculations the important parameters are listed in table 1. There is a trade off here between vertical stroke and horizontal resolution and in all cases the available force is not large. The main advantages lie in the response time, which for small capacitors will be very short, and the required energy as given by {4}.

$$\text{Energy } e = \tfrac{1}{2}CV^2 \qquad \{4\}$$

Given a 10 pF capacitive element driven from a 2000 Volt supply, an energy per cycle of 20 μJ can be expected. When vibrated at a frequency of 250 Hz [4] an average power of around 10 mW per element and a total power consumption of around 10 W can be expected from a 1000 element display.

Piezoelectric

The first tactile arrays constructed from piezoelectric bimorph actuators had limited vertical movement and required comparatively long actuator elements. Cutaneous stimulation was traditionally achieved by vibration of the element tip against the finger ends [10]. Though the spatial resolution can be very good the vertical movement was extremely limited. The frequency of the vibration may be changed to provide more information but it is hardly representative of physical hardness.

In the meantime developments in piezoelectric and electrostrictive device technology have made strokes of several millimetres possible which may further be increased by the use of mechanical [11] or hydraulic [12] amplification. Large quantity manufacture of very small bimorphic elements has lead to relatively small, cost effective pneumatic valves. One distinct advantage of piezoelectric elements is that, being capacitive, no sustaining energy is required. Once switched on they remain on until short circuited. Commercially available piezoelectric pneumatic and hydraulic valves are not yet small enough to allow the control of large area haptic displays. However, this is an area of technology which will be closely monitored in the immediate future.

The switch-on energy for a piezoelectric device can be calculated from {5}

$$\text{Energy} \quad e \; = \; \tfrac{1}{2}CV^2 \qquad \{5\}$$

Which for a 500 pF bimorph element powered from 200 Volts gives an energy of 10 µJ. Even when used in the vibratory mode this corresponds to no more than 10 µW. A 1000 element display would have a very modest power consumption of 10 mW.

Shape Memory Materials

Shape memory materials have the property of thermally reversible mechanical deformation. The commonest, NiTi (or similar) metal alloys, are known appropriately as shape memory alloys. Arrays for minimal invasive surgery applications have been built from devices comprising a shape memory alloy (SMA) spring and a normal metal return spring. As shown in table 1, strokes of 2 to 3 mm are typical and forces can be as high as 5N [13]. The main disadvantage is the response time. The electrical resistance being around 0.6 Ω means currents of several amps are required if rapid heating is desired. Power requirements of around 0.5 Watt per element means 500 W for a 1000 element array.

A rather lower power consumption (0.06 Watts per element) was recorded by Brenner and co-workers for a more complicated bistable device [14]. However the stroke is limited to less than 1 mm with a force of 350 mN and the response time is similarly slow, typically 3.4 seconds.

Shape memory polymers (SMP) have similar properties to SMA but for entirely different physical reasons. They have been used for the production of controllable topology surfaces, but hitherto not in discrete array formats [15]. Unfortunately they are also slow and suffer from the same thermal problems as SMA systems.

Electrostimulation

This is another method investigated by Bliss and Coworkers. By using a relatively high voltage but at the same time limiting the current to within safe boundaries, a small electric shock, just beyond the threshold of physical sensation, can be induced in the finger tips via each tactile element [10].

A 20µs wide pulses with 2 ms spacing gives an average duty cycle of 1%. For a 100 Volts pulse with a peak current of 10 mA an average power of 10 mW can be expected. A thousand elements would then require a maximum of 10 Watts.

Electrorheological

To reduce the scale of the devices being used one option is the employment of an active medium such as electrorheological fluids. ER fluids behave as normal Newtonian liquids until subjected to a high electric field strength (>2 kV/mm). Then they undergo a phase change from liquid to a quasi-solid state. This means that flow control can be achieved by simply passing the fluid between two electrodes. This makes the design of hydraulic valves extremely simply and their construction potentially very small.

Figure 4. 16 Element ERF tactile matrix.

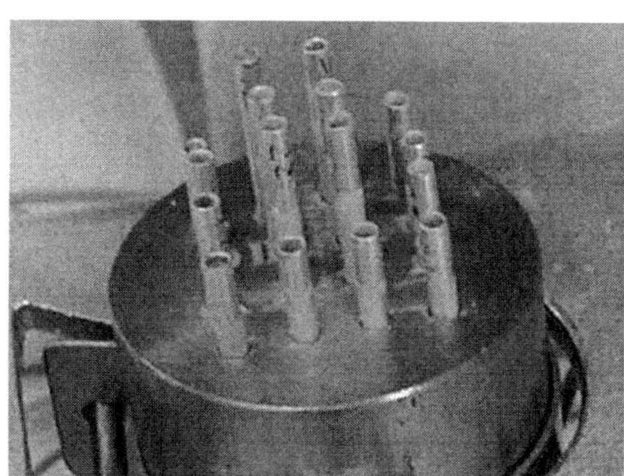

Another possibility is to switch the elements themselves with the ER fluid integrated into the tactile display directly. This has been done previously for binary (on/off) displays [5], and more recently with a degree of vertical resolution as shown in figure 4 [16].

Test results from two versions, one with cylindrical elements as shown in figure 4 and the other with planar elements, are shown in table 2.

Table 2. New electrorheological actuators used in tactile displays

Physical actuation method	Array size	Typical force	Horizontal resolution	Vertical stroke	Band-width	Power/ Element
Cylindrical	4 x 4	1.4 N	ca. 5 mm	30 mm	>20 Hz	ca. 20 mW
Planar	4 x 4	0.6 N	ca. 3 mm	40 mm	>20 Hz	ca. 27 mW

From table 2 it can be seen that electrorheological fluids enjoy a comparatively low power consumption. For a 1400 Volt device a maximum current of around 20 µA can be expected.

This gives a total power consumption under 30 Watts for a 1000 element array - a considerable energy saving when compared with hydraulic or electromagnetic systems.

A further advantage of electrorheology is the ability to build valves whose diameters are no wider than those of the hydraulic tubing. In fact, simple valves can be made by coating the insides of the hydraulic tubes with stripfilm electrodes. Combining the hydraulic cylinder array of figure 3 with such valves makes an electrically controllable hydraulic array without undue size overhead or extra power demands.

Micromachining fabrication methods

In order to achieve high spatial resolution, a single tactel is limited to a diameter of a few millimetres. This requires the application of modern fabrication methods. In addition to conventional drilling and milling, micromachining now offers a wider range of potential manufacturing techniques. Going from design to production, several methods, processes and materials can be used to produce micro structured products.

For the realisation of profiles by hot embossing or injection moulding it is necessary to produce mould inserts possessing the negative pattern of the final microstructure. Mould inserts can be produced for example by high precision milling for structure sizes down to 100 µm. Smaller structures can be realised using processes like Advanced Silicon Etching or LIGA-technology.

By using a special plasma etching technique it is possible to fabricate silicon structures independent of the crystal orientation with depths of several hundred micrometres and high aspect ratio. High density fluorine plasma is used to isotropically etch the silicon with high etching rates. To achieve almost vertical side walls in the range of 80°-90° the addition of monomer gases is necessary for side wall passivation. During the ASE-process, the alternation between a bias enhanced plasma etching step and a conformal deposition of a Teflon like polymer leads to a deep etch process with a high etching rate (several µm/min) and high anisotropy.

After successful fabrication of a mould insert different technologies for moulding can be used (Figure 5). The easiest way of achieving polymer micro structured components is the use of vacuum casting. First, a master structure must be fabricated by one of the above mentioned technologies. The master is embedded in a silicone rubber, which is then used as a mould for e.g. polyurethane (PUR) resin. PUR is a duroplast which is cured at 60 °C for 2 hours. This technique allows the fabrication of a limited number of parts in a short time and is therefore often used for rapid prototyping. However, large scale mass production is not normally possible due to the limited lifetime of the silicone moulds.

The two main moulding processes for the replication of micro components are injection moulding and hot embossing. Using hot embossing it is possible to save high costs during the development stage because only a mould insert together with a simple demoulding construction are needed. Nevertheless, it is possible to achieve high aspect ratios and stress-free results because of short flow paths and slow moulding speeds. Different polymer materials like PMMA, COC or POM are well suited to realising such prototypes.

For higher volume production, injection moulding offers advantages over hot embossing processes. The polymer melt is injected with high pressure into the cavity with the microstructured mould insert. After the polymer is solidified, the tool is opened and the moulded parts are automatically ejected. For each product the construction of an appropriate tool is necessary. This includes a nozzle, the *runner system* for the distribution of the melt into the cavities, ejection pins, heating and cooling circuits and precise guide posts. The higher tool costs are more than compensated for by shorter cycle times and the possibility of a fully automated process. The choice of materials includes practically all thermoplasts and if reaction injection moulding is used, certain elastomers and duroplasts can also be utilised. Compared to the conventional injection moulding process, micro injection moulding differs in some aspects. Firstly, inhomogeneous heating systems have to be applied to improve the filling of small structures. Secondly, in many cases the mould cavity can be evacuated before the polymer melt is injected.

Figure 5. Three microstructure moulding processes.

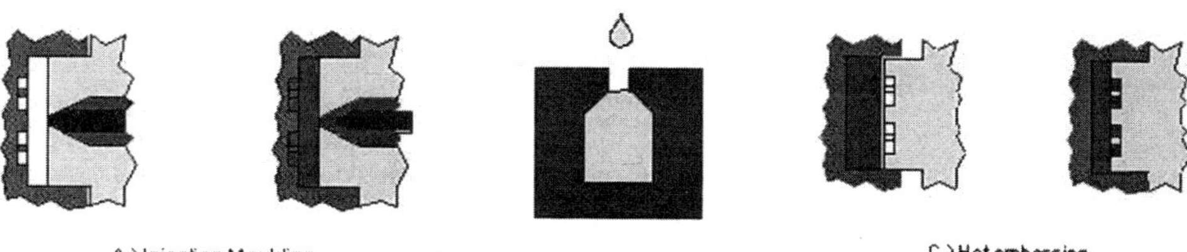

Medical safety aspects and classification

Such parameters as accuracy, repeatability and resolution must be known to within defined tolerances for all equipment used for instrumentation and measurement purposes - also over predetermined lifetimes. In addition to general mechanical, electrical, thermal, acoustic and ergonomic design criteria, other factors such as electromagnetic, material and chemical compatibility must be considered.

For the potential market development of such a system consideration must be given to the guidelines of the European regulations for Medical products [93/94/EWG]. Safety aspects should be addressed early during the development stage. Difficulties identified at this point can then be corrected in a timely manner thus saving much greater costs should such problems be discovered later.

Depending on the level of threat to life and safety and technical risk factors, medical products are divided into four classes (I, IIa, IIb and III). A haptically explorable array is a display unit for the surgeon or medical practitioner and patients would not normally be expected to come into contact with it. Consequently, like virtually all non-invasive medical instruments, such a system would fall into class I. This means that general safety aspects are the responsibility of the manufacturer and intensive testing for type approval is not normally necessary. Nevertheless, before the product is brought into commercial use it must conform to the laws governing medical equipment and posses the necessary CE markings and the appropriate user documentation.

Spare parts and consumables are also governed by the same classification. For example the electrorheological fluid, if sold separately, must also meet the same type approval as the equipment with which it is to be used. Under the same regulations, medical products under class I may not include materials which are classified as drugs or medicines under [65/65/EWG]. Computer software, in this case necessary for display control, also falls under the same classification as the hardware it is used with.

Other aspects to be considered are: Choice of materials used - toxicity, flammability etc., minimisation of risk though fire and explosion with old or defective equipment, mechanical and electrical design for the reduction of general injury risks.

Conclusions

Many electromechanical techniques exist for the potential production of haptically explorable arrays for the tactile presentation of elastographic images. The choice of design depends heavily on the size of the array and the desired resolution. The method of switching is most important as in many cases the switch or valve is larger than the tactile elements themselves. The exception is electrorheological fluid based systems. Here there are other problems as high voltages must be switched. This is no mean feat and is another major task within this project.

Finally, whichever array system is used, it must be interfaced with the ultrasound sensor system and the entire control carried out by software. This will be done by presenting data in MatLab™ format which will be used to drive control algorithms written in LabView™. Of course the system is not restricted to use with elastograms. Other images such as standard video, x-ray, infra-red etc., could be just as easily displayed.

References

[1] Pesavento, A.; Lorenz, A.; Ermert, H.: System for real-time elastography. *Electronics Letters*, vol. 35, no. 11, 941-942, 27th May 1999

[2] Scheipers, U.; Pesavento, A.; Lorenz, A.; Ermert, H.; Sommerfeld, H.-J.; Garcia-Schürmann, M.; Kühne, K.; Senge T.; Philippou S.: Ultrasonic multifeature tissue characterization for the early detection of prostate cancer. *IEEE Ultrasonics Symposium*, 1265-1268, 2001

[3] Rogers. C.H. - Choice of stimulator frequency for tactile arrays - *IEEE Trans. Man-Mchine Systems* - vol MMS-11, No. 1, 5-11, March 1970

[4] Verillo. R.T - Subjective magnitude functions for tactovibration - *IEEE Trans. Man-Mchine Systems* - vol MMS-11, No. 1, 19-24, March 1970

[5] Monkman G.J. - An Electrorheological Tactile Display - *Presence* (Journal of Teleoperators and Virtual Environments) - Vol. 1, issue 2, 219-228, MIT Press, July 1992

[6] Seeley H.F. & J.C. Bliss - Compenstory tracking with visual and tactile dispalys - *IEEE Trans. Human Factors in Electronics* - vol HFE-7, 84-90, June 1966

[7] Festo - Einfachwirkender Zylinder EG-2,5 - Festo Pneumatik, p1.2/20-1, Europa-Programm 1998

[8] Collins C.C. - Tactile Television: Mechnical and electrical image projection - *IEEE Trans. Man-Mchine Systems* - vol MMS-11, No. 1, 65-71, March 1970

[9] Kämper K.P., W. Ehrfeld, B. Hagemann, H. Lehr, F. Michel, A. Schirling, Ch. Thuringen & Th. Wittig - Electromagnetic permanent magnet micromotor with integrated micro gear box - *5th Interntional conf. On new Actuators*, 429-432 - Bremen, June 1996

[10] Bliss J.C., M.H. Katcher, C.H. Rogers & R.P. Shepard - Optical to tactile imge conversion for the blind - *IEEE Trans. Man-Mchine Systems* - vol MMS-11, No. 1, 58-65, March 1970

[11] Salim. R & H. Wurmus - Multi gearing compliant mechanisms for piezoelectric actuated microgrippers - *Actuator'98: 6th Internatonal Conference on New Actuators*, 186-188 - Messe Bremen GmbH, Bremen, June 1998

[12] Scheunemann. M, & H. Widmann - Tactile actuators for tactile feedbck systems - *6th Interntional conf. On new Actuators*, 333-336 - Bremen, June 1998

[13] Fischer. H, R. Trapp & B. Hoffmann - Actuator array for use in minimal invasive surgery - *5th Interntional conf. On new Actuators*, 383-337 - Bremen, June 1996

[14] Brenner W., S. Mitic, A. Vujanic & G. Popovic - Micro-actuation principles for high-resolution graphic tactile displays - *7th Interntional conf. On new Actuators*, 567-570 - Bremen, June 2000

[15] Monkman G.J. - Controllable Shape Retention - *Journal of Intelligent Materials Systems & Structures* - Vol 5, No. 4, 567-575, July 1994

[16] Böse. H, G. J. Monkman, H. Freimuth, D. Klein, H. Ermert, M. Baumann, S. Egersdörfer, O. T. Bruhns - ER Fluid Based Haptic System for Virtual Reality - *8th Interntional conf. On new Actuators*, 351-354 - Bremen, June 2002

Acknowledgements

The authors would like to gratefully acknowledge the BMBF for financial support and the administrative and engineering workshop staff at the Fachhochschule Regensburg for their valuable assistance.

Address for correspondence

Professor Dr. Gareth J. Monkman
Fachhochschule Regensburg - University of Applied Sciences
Fachbereich Elektrotechnik
Prüfeninger Strasse 58, 93049 Regensburg, Germany
phone: +49 941 943 1108
fax: +49 941 943 1424
e.mail: gareth.monkman@e-technik.fh-regensburg.de

Cybercare NDMS: An Improved Strategy for Biodefense Using Information Technologies

JOSEPH M. ROSEN, ELIOT GRIGG, SUSAN MC GRATH,
SCOTT LILLIBRIDGE, C. EVERETT KOOP

*Dartmouth-Hitchcock Medical Center, Department of Plastic Surgery,
One Hospital Drive, Lebanon, NH 03756, USA*

Abstract. The National Disaster Medical System (NDMS) was created in the early 1980's, and it was designed to meet the threats of the time. Today the threats are much less discreet and predictable. They are distributed; they move and spread quickly; and they walk silently among us. Specifically, biological agents are an enemy unlike any we have had to deal with before. They offer unique challenges that fly in the face of current doctrine. We must redesign the NDMS in order to contain and eliminate this new threat. Tools exist today capable of effectively coordinating distributed resources – even through containment borders. We need to strengthen our public health system, create a net-centric disaster management system, and blur the boundaries between local and federal resources. Ultimately we must move from an incremental, echelon-based response to an immediate, continuous response. This can be accomplished by adding inexpensive, well-established information technologies to the existing response system.

Problem

A Brief History of NDMS: The National Disaster Medical System (NDMS) was created in the early 1980's. A series of hurricanes and earthquakes in the 1960's and '70's had focused attention on the issue of natural disasters and brought about increased legislation. In 1978, the Department of Defense (DOD) staged a worldwide deployment exercise called Nifty Nugget, which revealed a lack of flexibility when multiple transportation modes – air, land, and sea – were required. In addition, various data processing systems could not function together. Unity of command was impossible because no single commander had overall responsibility and authority to coordinate and direct the use of various available transport capabilities. President Carter's 1979 executive order merged many of the separate disaster-related responsibilities into a new Federal Emergency Management Agency (FEMA). Finally, in 1983 FEMA, the Department of Health and Human Services (HHS), the Department of Defense (DOD), and the Department of Veterans Affairs (VA) came together to create the NDMS. FEMA supplied disaster response teams and management, HHS contributed medical supplies, DOD was in charge of evacuation, and VA offered vacant hospital beds and doctors around the country.

The NDMS was designed to meet the threats of the time. Natural and transportation disasters looked much the same as they do today. Terrorism, however, looked very different 20 years ago. In 1975 a number of bombings in New York City were attributed to the Puerto Rican National Liberation Army, and a few people were killed. In '82 a bomb exploded on a Pan Am flight in Hawaii, and several people were injured. In 1983, the U.S.

Marine Barracks in Beirut were attacked by a truck filled with explosives and 241 soldiers were killed. While the losses were tragic, all of the events were similar. They all involved conventional explosives. They were all contained within specific geographic areas and did not threaten infrastructure. They all had discreet beginning and end points regardless of when first responders arrived. As a result, all of these events made the nightly news, but none ever threatened American living rooms.

Preparing for such threats, the National Disaster Medical system is designed by concentrating highly trained personnel with sophisticated resources, called Disaster Medical Assistance Teams (DMATs), and positioning them strategically around the country. In the event of a disaster, teams are dispatched to the crisis area. Upon arrival, they provide triage, austere medical care, and casualty clearing/staging. The larger the disaster, the more DMATs are dispatched. But integrating with local resources has always been a challenge. The DMATs cannot possibly train with every local emergency system. Because local healthcare resources are often overwhelmed by the sudden influx of casualties, the NDMS is designed to evacuate 90% of casualties to remote facilities while treating only 10% on-scene. Transportation is under the auspices of the DOD, and primarily comes in the form of aeromedical evacuation. While concern about large-scale disasters, like earthquakes, led to the creation of the NDMS, even earthquakes – with their potential for numerous casualties – are fundamentally different from the challenges we face today.

21st Century Threats

While conventional explosives will probably still be involved in the majority of terrorist incidents today, new threats and possibilities have arisen that present very differently from what we are accustomed to. As technological, political, and social barriers disappear, a world of Weapons of Mass Destruction (WMDs) has become the focus of national security. The most unusual and potentially destructive of these weapons is the family of biological weapons. Biological agents are much more insidious than conventional explosives; people are infected silently.

Unlike chemical weapons they spread from person to person indefinitely. They are even more psychologically damaging than nuclear weapons. They are also unique in that they will encounter the public health system long before the emergency response system – spreading quietly until someone notices. And that's the simple version. A creative terrorist would deploy distributed, sequenced bio-attacks in conjunction with a cyber-attack to take down our information infrastructure.

The World Trade Center Attack on 9/11 was a *tactical* attack. Thousands of people lost their lives, but our society as a whole was never in danger. It shocked the nation, but it was not a *strategic* attack. The impact of a tactical attack is measured by the amount of physical damage done: the number of lives lost, property damaged, total economic impact. Tactical attacks affect the outcomes of battles. Strategic attacks affect the outcomes of wars. Strategic attacks affect economies, infrastructures, and mass psychology. Strategic attacks overturn momentum, sway politics and change strategies. When a WMD becomes a strategic weapon, it becomes a Disruptive Mission Weapon (DMW). In a strategic conflict, the number of casualties alone is not the measure of success. Twenty-five cities in America each with 200 people infected with a biological agent are much more disruptive than 5000 casualties at the World Trade Center. The potential destructive power of biological weapons is much greater than that of a plane commandeered by suicidal terrorists. Between the casualties, the terror, and the economic losses they can inflict, biological weapons have the potential to overcome the will of the nation.

In the last few years exercises like TOPOFF, Dark Winter and ones performed at Dartmouth have demonstrated that our current disaster response system is ill-prepared for biological terrorism [2,3,4,11]. Like Nifty Nugget did in the late 1970's these exercises must elicit change in the way we do business. We must improve upon the current NDMS model to better address the unique threat presented by biological terrorism.

Biological weapons with their unique characteristics affect the overall disaster response strategy in a number of ways. The most damaging aspect of biological weapons is their ability to spread throughout a population after the initial dispersal. The tempo of the disease can dictate the difference between a tactical and a strategic attack. Therefore, the single most important aspect of response to a bio-weapon is to control the spread. Control requires: (1) early detection, (2) rapid response, and ultimately (3) containment. Because early detection is critical, and because bio-casualties will first surface in the public health system, the public health system itself must be enhanced rather than simply being augmented by DMATs that drop in after an attack is discovered.

In the event of a true bio-disaster, containment will be necessary, and containment dramatically changes the rules of disaster response. It is worth noting that containment – the enforced, physical isolation of a geographic area – will necessarily require reverse-containment. Nothing capable of carrying the disease is allowed to leave the "hot zone" for fear that it may be infected. At the same time, nothing capable of becoming infected is allowed to enter the hot zone from outside. So, not only can patients not be evacuated from the hot zone to remote healthcare facilities, but responders cannot enter into the hot zone (unless they are equipped with the most sophisticated gear and thoroughly decontaminated). But for the most part, human resources and casualties – at least to the extent that would be necessary in a major disaster – will not be able to cross the border.

Infected patients still need medical attention. The hot zone still needs a huge amount of medical resources. And commanders outside the hot zone must keep track of what is happening inside. There is hope. Containment means that things capable of harboring the disease cannot cross the border; things that cannot possibly carry the disease, however, may travel as they please. Fortunately, there are a number of unexploited resources capable of doing just that.

Concept

Changing the Mission of NDMS: While Project Bioshield is an important step in creating effective countermeasures against biological agents, it is only a piece of an overall strategy. Countermeasures target specific agents, but in this age of biotechnology we cannot predict what organisms will be used against us. Therefore we need a strategy capable of defending against *any and all* threats. At the same time, we do not want to revamp the entire existing disaster response system. It is important to leverage what resources and structures are already in place. We want to involve the resources of FEMA, HHS, DOD and VA like the DMATs or the 80,000 VA hospital beds ready to respond. Finally, the cost of the new system will be small and will make use of established information technologies used for years in the academic and business arenas.

The major change for the NDMS is a mission change, and the major cost will be for training. From a medical point of view, a bio-event is a relatively simple affair for no other reason than there are very few medical interventions available to us. Treatment primarily involves pharmaceuticals, supportive therapy and, most importantly, isolation. Complex surgical teams, sterile environments, and sophisticated imaging equipment – that may be needed for crush or burn patients – are not required.

Logistically, on the other hand, a bio-event is a nightmare because the clock is always ticking, movement of resources is restricted, and tempo wins the war. We must combine the goals of casualty management, surge-capacity and containment into a single goal: stopping the spread of the disease. We must bridge the artificial divide between crisis and consequence management to form a coherent effort. We must balance the specialization of resources with the distribution of resources. We must improve the actions and systems of the NDMS to effectively address the biological threat.

Paradigm Shifts

There are 5 major paradigm shifts that must occur in the NDMS in order to meet the challenges of the 21st century.

Response Strategy (Tempo)

The philosophy of incremental response must be replaced by immediate response. The slow accumulation of resources as a crisis develops will likely not be quick enough to contain a biological outbreak [2,3,4,11]. Today local resources encounter a disaster first, and then they are supported by incoming federal resources after a state of emergency is declared. By the time a crisis is detected, the scale of it is appreciated, and federal resources are put into play, it may be too late.

Figure 1. Current, Incremental Response Requirements

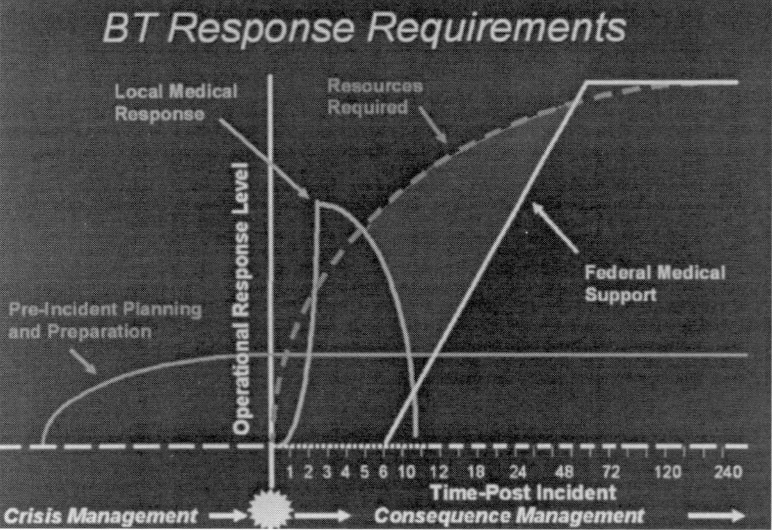

Rather than a two-step process, disaster response should be a singular effort from local, state, regional, and federal resources combined using information technologies.

Figure 2. Future, Integrated Response Requirements

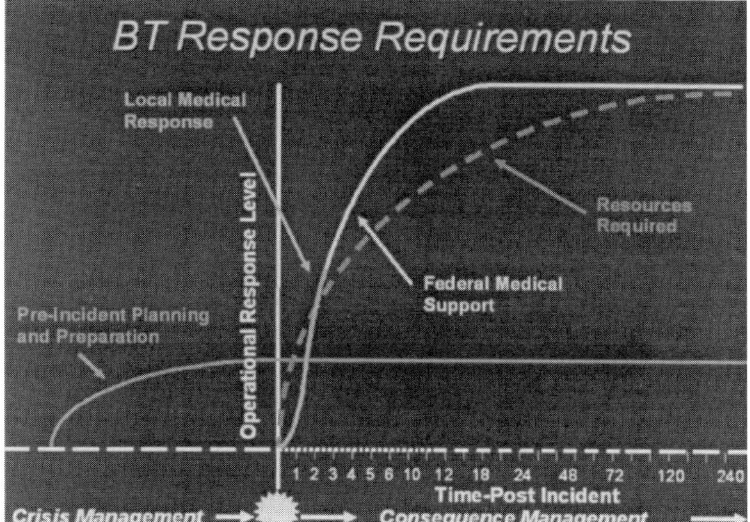

Care Model (Telemedicine)

Isolation must replace evacuation as the primary goal of patient management in a bio-event. Evacuation was designed to lessen the burden on local hospitals that are already operating near or at capacity. But now everyone must be treated locally. Without evacuation, patients must be accommodated somewhere besides the hospitals. In fact, we don't want to concentrate patients in the hospitals anyway where they will infect everyone else there. This does not necessarily mean that specially sealed isolation rooms have to be constructed for each patient either; that's logistically unrealistic. We will discuss just where exactly we will accommodate these patients later in the paper when we discuss the use of facilities. Suffice to say, everyone already has somewhere to sleep at night that is designed for privacy. A little creative shuffling of available resources will come into play. Without evacuation, more than just beds will be in short supply. Healthcare personnel and medical supplies will also have to be augmented without breaking containment. This is the classic problem of healthcare surge-capacity.

Similar to the incremental response problem, the standard in disaster medicine is echelon-based care. A patient is transported from one level of care to the next with different providers at each location, little management in transit, and ultimately discontinuous care. A better model is continuous care where patients are followed by single or distinct groups of providers throughout the system. Without physical transportation and with the network-centric system described later, this form of care will be possible. Data will flow when patients cannot, and as a result care will be more consistent and uninterrupted.

Connectivity (Situational Awareness)

Connectivity will be the buzzword of 21st century disaster response. Everyone involved in the response – from first responders to healthcare facilities to command and control – must be connected in an efficient, pervasive, redundant way. This will allow for the distribution of resources, effective communication, situational awareness, inter-agency coordination, and action across borders. Connectivity is the backbone of the entire envisioned system, and it directly facilitates the next two paradigm shifts. Connectivity is important within the hot zone to coordinate response efforts, but it is equally important between the hot and cold zones. Electrons can pass through the containment border, and that simple principle can save the isolated community from total "isolation".

Characteristics of the network itself will be further explored in the Network section. Combining the care model with connectivity we create a new patient flow for the NDMS. Rather than being physically evacuated, patients are virtually evacuated (Figure3). The same doctors that would oversee the patients at remote VA hospitals are now electronically connected to local casualties to manage their care. The first responders act as the physical healthcare presence. They locate, identify, and triage patients; and, according to physicians' recommendations, perform treatment. The red elements in Figure 3 highlight the info-tech additions to the existing system.

Figure 3. New NDMS Patient Flow Diagram

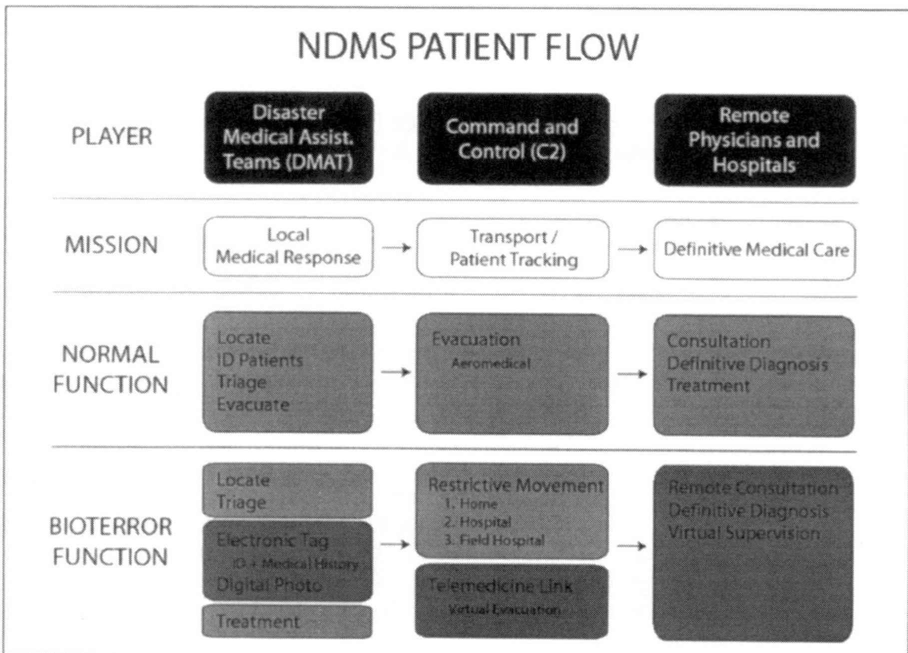

Distributed (Cyber-Structure)

As connectivity becomes more pervasive, the physical (or platform) based structure must be de-emphasized while the cyber (or information) based structure must be emphasized. Again, information flows when patients cannot.

A cyber-based structure allows for a network-centric approach. The network-centric approach has been a major component of military infrastructures in recent years; however this was not always the case. The C2 model that governed military operations for many years was platform-based, meaning that individual nodes were largely responsible for sensing, recognizing, and attacking the enemy. A platform in the military context can range in size from a soldier to an aircraft to a ship, but fundamentally a platform is an entity equipped with organic sensors and weapons with one or more warfighters in the loop making critical decisions. The inability of platforms to share information, except through a remote C2 unit, leads to limited situational awareness and sub-optimal performance. Platforms that can share information and leverage the assets (sensors or weapons) of other isolated platforms are more aware, more flexible, and consequently more capable.

The platform-based warfare model has given way to a network-centric warfare (NCW) model based on the recognition that a well informed, geographically dispersed fighting force is more effective than a concentrated, isolated force. In this new model, shown in Figure 4, platforms share information to increase their accuracy and coordination. Our healthcare practitioners are akin to independent platforms, collecting and sharing data, and providing services locally and remotely. Under normal conditions, the network enables collaboration of health care practitioners across geographically dispersed locations, and in mass casualty situations, incident command centers can be added to the network with situational awareness applications that allow them to effectively manage the crisis.

One way to understand how the net-centric structure works is to trace an entity as it moves through such a system. To begin with, imagine talking on a cell phone while driving in a car (not the best idea, but imagine nonetheless). Each cellular tower is a platform; they transmit and receive signals in a geographic area. The cell phone is also a platform picking up voice and sending and receiving to the tower. However, as the cell phone moves around it jumps from tower to tower depending up which has the strongest signal. All of the towers are on a signal network so that each knows which tower is closest to the cell phone and should make the wireless connection. Despite the movement of the cell phone the connection to the network is maintained and the conversation is coherent.

Now imagine a naval war theatre with a number of platforms: Aegis cruisers, satellites, and C2 airplanes (Figure 4). The Aegis cruiser has command and control capability, sensors and weapons. The C2 airplane has command and control and sensors. The satellite has only sensors. A missile fired from an Aegis cruiser begins its journey under the control of the cruiser. In mid-flight control is transferred to the satellite as the original cruiser moves farther away. Towards the end, the C2 plane flying directly over the target takes over control until impact. Situational awareness is enhanced throughout the system.

Figure 4. Network-Centric Warfare

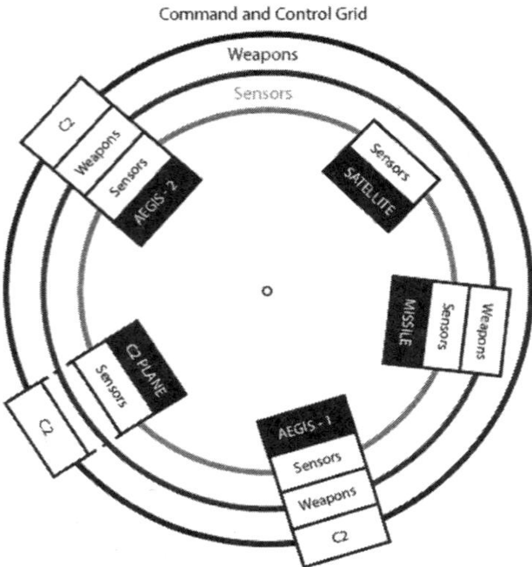

Now imagine a patient moving from the scene of a train wreck to a triage facility to an ambulance to a tertiary care facility. All the while sensors on the patient are collecting physiological data that is being wirelessly transmitted – via various means along the way – to the network. Medical information entered at each stage is also entered into the system. When the patient arrives at the tertiary care facility, surgeons have been monitoring the patient en route and have all of his medical history since extrication from the train on hand.

Figure 5. Network-Centric Healthcare

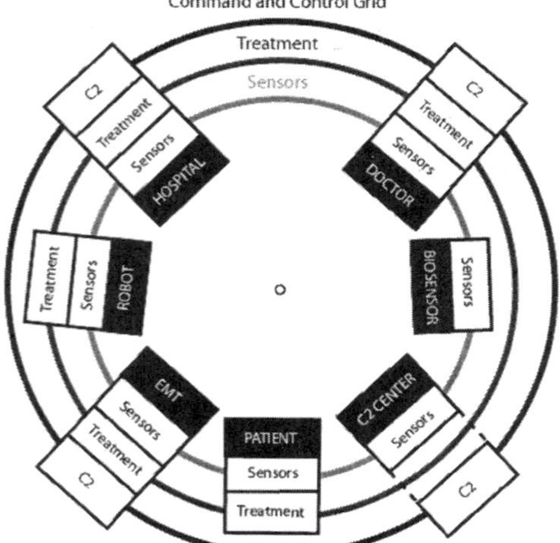

Command and Control

Detailed command and control (C2) must be combined with *mission* command and control. "The first response to uncertainty is to try to minimize it by creating a powerful, highly efficient command and control apparatus able to process huge amounts of information and intended to reduce nearly all unknowns. The result is *detailed* command and control. Such a system stems from the belief that if we can impose order and certainty on the disorderly and uncertain battlefield, then successful results are predictable" [8]. Detailed C2 is coercive; it maintains control by personal direction or detailed directive. It is highly centralized and formal. Detailed command and control emphasizes vertical, linear information flow: in general, information flows up the chain of command and orders flow down. This is the standard for C2 today.

Figure 6. Detailed Command and Control

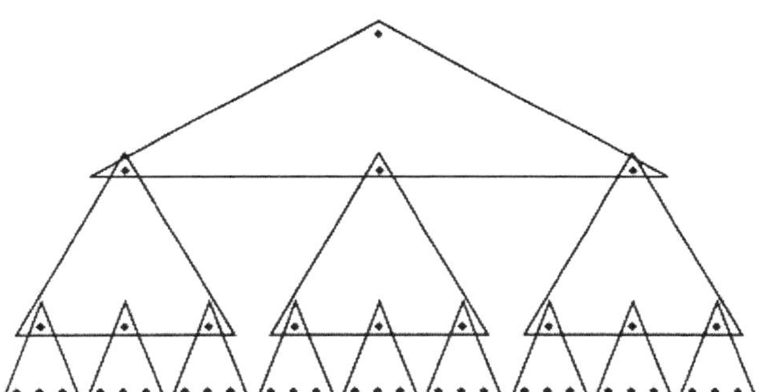

"*Mission* command and control accepts the turbulence and uncertainty of war. Rather than increase the level of certainty that we seek, by mission command and control we reduce the degree of certainty that we need. Mission command and control can be described as *spontaneous*. ... Subordinates are guided not by detailed instructions and control measures but by their knowledge of the requirements of the overall mission" [8]. Mission C2 decentralizes decision-making authority and grants subordinates significant freedom of action. It is much more informal and flexible than detailed C2. It increases tempo and improves the ability to deal with fluid and disorderly situations. It relies more on implicit communication so it is less vulnerable to disruption from a loss of communication lines. In addition, because it requires less communication to be sent up and down the chain of command it is less prone to the effects of delay and distortion.

Figure 7. Mission Command and Control

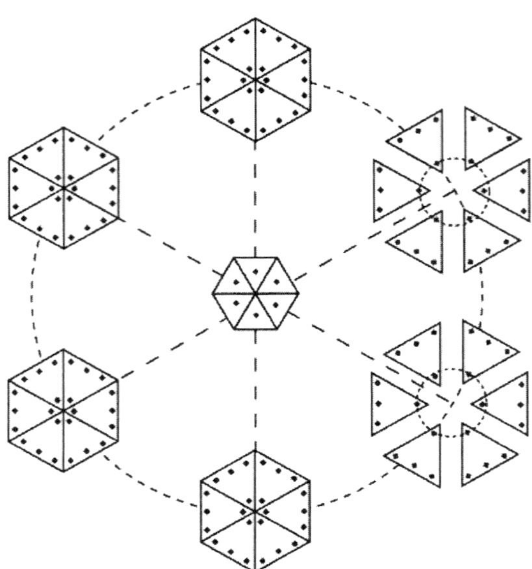

In the environment of uncertainty, complexity, and variability, mission C2 encourages judgment, creativity, and initiative. Orders are task-oriented; commanders must communicate the *intent* of the mission rather than detailed, step-by-step instructions. In reality, the ideal command structure is a combination of the two:

Figure 8. Combined Command and Control

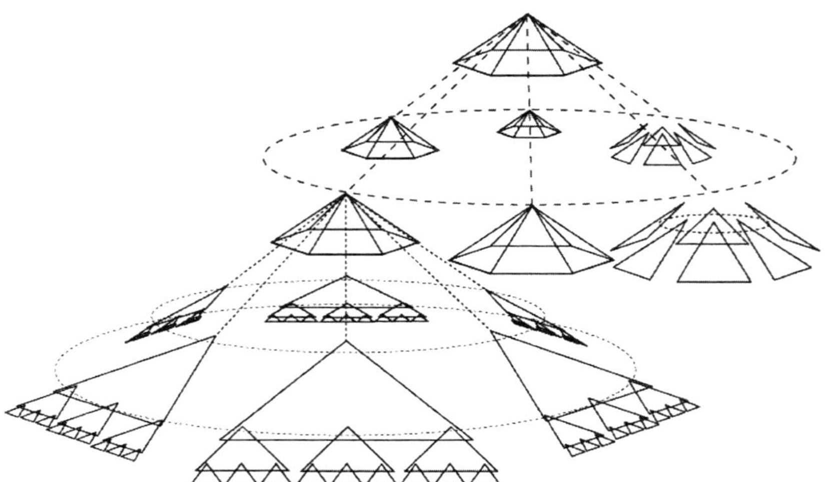

Mission C2 is appropriate at the highest levels where the operation is too complex to keep close tabs on. At intermediate levels, commanders are put in charge of overall tasks – like securing a specific area – and the lowest level of command actually completes the task with detailed C2. The command space is a shared environment where distributed C2 centers act together. For a more thorough discussion of C2 strategies and technologies see [5].

Cybercare Concept

Cybercare is information intensive co-ordination. Instantaneous and unaware of spatial distances, cyberspace allows local and federal resources to function in synchrony rather than alongside one another. The future of response to biological disasters is a fusion of creative, grass-roots utilization of available resources within a containment area and advanced cyber-technologies connecting distributed resources within and without. As it exists today, the National Disaster Medical System is essentially a patient regulation and dissemination scheme. In the future, the NDMS will be a net-centric, telemedicine system based on advanced networking technologies that combine all levels of the response structure into a single, distributed entity capable of mobilizing a nationwide, near-instantaneous response while maintaining containment.

In order to realize the cybercare system in a relevant way, the 5 paradigm shifts need to be woven into the 4 phases of disaster response:

1. Preparation
2. Detection
3. Control
4. Treatment

In doing so we will describe in detail the practical components of the cybercare system in the next section.

System Components

Preparation: There are 4 stages of preparation: (1) planning, (2) education, (3) training, and (4) mobilization.

Planning is the process of taking stock of what resources are available and then speculating how they would best be implemented in the event of a disaster. Planning is usually overseen by small committees given the task of formulating a disaster plan. As the foundation of future operations, the planning phase must elicit input from the variety of players in disaster response.

Education is informing everyone else about what the plan contains or other information relevant to disaster preparation. In a hospital it might involve updating the staff of changes in the disaster plan or making sure all physicians are familiar with the clinical presentations of biological agents. We mention this step because disaster plans too often sit on shelves collecting dust while their contents never make it to the end-users.

Training is the most important part of preparing for a disaster. In order to be useful training has to be realistic – "train like you fight, fight like you train". It's true in the military; it's true in sports; and it's true for the healthcare system. The most simplistic way of accomplishing this is by making everyday tasks similar to those in a disaster. For example, using the same computers and interfaces that one does in everyday tasks. Another option is embedded training. An Automatic External Defibrillator is a simple example.

While largely automated, it trains the user where to place the pads and when to press the button during an actual event. A more complex treatment of just-in-time training of healthcare personnel will come in the Personnel section of the paper.

Simulation opens up exciting new opportunities for training. Simulation allows the construction of elaborate scenarios that are not feasible in reality due to cost, safety or scale. However, simulation's most exciting ability is to blend fiction with reality and training with operations. If a simulation is high enough fidelity then it can emulate reality in the ultimate "train like you fight" scenario. An air force pilot flying a Predator drone in practice uses the same joystick and interfaces that he does in real combat. In fact, the pilot may not be able to tell the difference. This quality can make the training more relevant and serious, prepare the soldier for the real event, and make the real event less stressful.

Figure 9. Integrated, Network-Centric Simulation

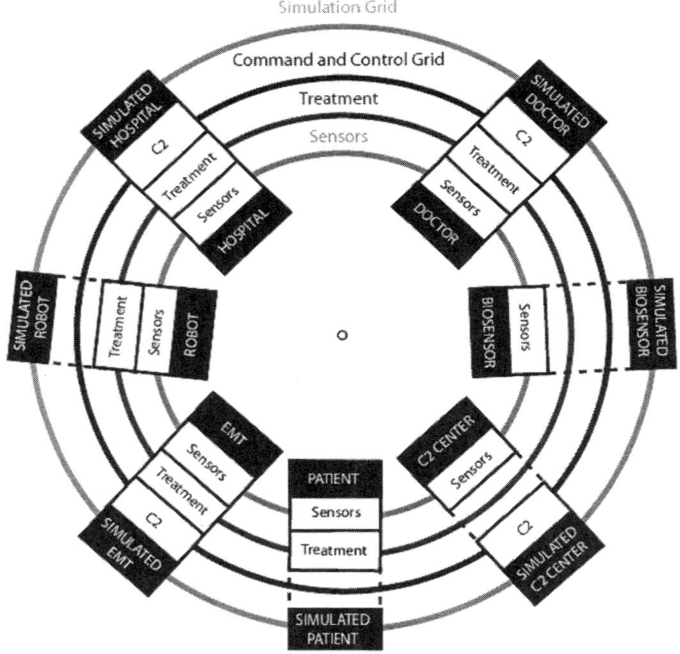

Simulation also has predictive value. They can be run to examine a number of possible outcomes, test interventions, and help to formulate disaster plans. Even during a disaster, a faster-than-real-time simulation can examine a situation, postulate possible outcomes from certain action, and serve as a decision support.

Training has historically been confined to individual organizations. A real disaster is a multi-agency operation requiring sophisticated (and sometimes chaotic) communication and coordination. Inter-agency training is crucial. The pitfalls of ignoring inter-agency training were tragically demonstrated on September 11 [9].

Finally, there has been some debate about the feasibility and utility of training everyone in the country as a first responder. While this is the ultimate goal of a truly distributed healthcare system with blanket coverage and less of a distinction between sophisticated federal and basic local resources, its particular incarnation is unclear. Ultimately such a basis of training could serve as the foundation of massive public health mobilizations in the event of a major disaster. A trained public could also increase the effectiveness of connecting healthcare professionals from the cold zone because they would have better trained local actors to operate through.

Mobilization itself is the most often neglected part of preparation. Mobilization is an act of political will usually in response to a perceived urgency. Mobilization can involve the military, industry, civil defense, or international alliances. As we are writing this paper the US military is mobilizing resources in the Persian Gulf region in preparation for war with Iraq. Troops are being stationed, ships are deployed, and negotiations are being made with local airbases. America has a history of assuming that conflict is transitory, avoidable, and outside US borders and so fails to properly mobilize until a crisis is well underway. With a bioevent, where time is critical, mobilization once the disaster begins will be too late. Federal, state, and local emergency response mechanisms must mobilize their resources. The public health sector must mobilize. And the American people must mobilize.

Detection

Detection begins with the public health system because that is where infected people will first appear. Today some areas are already monitoring inpatient records or emergency department visits for irregular patterns. As more patient records become electronic and data mining techniques grow more sophisticated with artificial intelligence, surveillance will become a powerful tool for recognizing suspicious trends. The key is to connect all of these systems in a coherent way so that a nation-wide picture of high resolution can be formed. Various inputs streams of different types and from different locations must be connected together. Humans are valuable sensors; physicians and the general public must be educated on how to identify suspicious symptoms.

Unfortunately people have to be sick enough to report to their doctor before they enter the healthcare system. Ideally detection should occur even earlier. A number of biotech companies are attempting to develop deployable biosensors. The military has been using handheld chemical sensors for years, but unfortunately biosensors are a little more complicated being essentially portable laboratories. An ideal biosensor should be small, portable, cost-effective, renewable, accurate, and specific. For the earliest detection they would be deployed around major metropolitan areas. Unfortunately they will only be effective if the bioagent is dispersed in the area – as opposed to brought in covertly by an infected individual. Still a cheap, portable, reliable biodetector would greatly shorten the turnaround time for laboratory confirmation, which today can only occur at the CDC or USAMRIID.

A variation on the patient record surveillance scheme is the sentinel node system. A model implementation is in the public school system. Like patient records, the system would monitor school attendance and look for abnormalities but pay particular attention to those individuals who rarely or never are absent, the "sentinel nodes". Baseline surveillance is limited, but the loss of a sentinel node would raise the fidelity of the surveillance for a closer inspection. The bottom line is that detection is critical in the world of bioresponse. Biological agents can easily be mistaken for common illnesses. The earlier detection, the earlier and faster a response is initiated, and the greater the odds are of controlling an outbreak.

Control

The Network: The entire system will be network-centric as described above. Information entered at any point in the network will have to travel to the appropriate location on the network in a seamless way. Remote physicians will connect to first responders; sensors will connect to the network; and commanders will receive inputs from everywhere.

Command resources will be distributed, so connections between them must be redundant, reliable, and fault tolerant. One way of dealing with data transmission over a volatile network is to use mobile agents. A mobile agent is the most general form of mobile code, namely, an executing program that can move at times of its own choosing from one machine to another. A mobile agent often, but not always, displays some of the other characteristics associated with agents, such as autonomy and adaptivity. Mobile agents are used to move computation to more attractive network locations, often to avoid the use of unreliable or low-bandwidth network links. Mobile agents are also used to autonomously filter and transport data from remote locations with the aim of saving bandwidth and increasing the timeliness of the data being delivered. A more extensive discussion of mobile agents and the rationale behind their use can be found in [1].

The system will use various network modalities. Many homes and businesses have access to the World Wide Web today. Internet2 will allow for more sophisticated connections between academic institutions. Wireless technologies are particularly important for their flexibility, omnipresence, and ease of installation. Wireless may come in the form of a Local Area Network (LAN) established to cover a given area, or satellite connections to access remote areas.

Global Positioning (GPS) and Geographic Information Systems (GIS) will be important throughout the network to keep track of the locations of patients and resources. The network will have to negotiate with a variety of sensors from biological agent detectors to physiological sensors. Security technologies will also be important, and their functions are described in the next section.

Telecare Nodes

Emergency Operations Centers (EOC) will be seamlessly connected from the federal level to the local level to one another and overseen by the NDMS Federal Coordinating Centers (FCC). The ideal command center is isolated from any bio-disaster by both space and time; one example is an Aegis cruiser that has been at sea for at least 2 weeks (the latency period of smallpox). There will be numerous command centers spread throughout the country so that no single one is necessary to maintain control, and the loss of any one will not impact the effectiveness of the others. All of the command centers come together in a virtual command space called a Virtual Operations Center (VOC). Using teleimmersion technologies commanders will be able to enter and leave VOCs instantaneously. Different levels of command will only be able to view what they have access to. They will be able to interact with 3-dimensional models based on real-time data from the field. Manipulation and presentation of the data will occur in user-friendly ways that would be physically impossible in the physical world.

Their primary functions include: (1) critical care tracking, (2) medical surveillance, (3) incident and event management, (4) data retrieval, and (5) collaboration and teleimmersion. Specifically incident and event management requires: mission C2, communication, coordination, situational awareness, and reachback. Individual missions vary by command center location and type. At the federal level they will oversee to overall progress and coordination of response agencies and efforts. In the hot zone command centers will integrate incoming resources with local resources and ensure that a detailed, accurate picture of the hot zone is portrayed to higher levels of command. Specifically hospitals will input information about the movement and status of patients and medical resources. In the cold zone command centers will continually monitor for new attacks and manage cold zone issues like panic management and media relations. Alternatively they will offset the cognitive load of hot zone C2 centers with brain or computing power because they are seamlessly connected on the network with the same access to information as the centers in the hot zone. Hospitals in the cold zone will specifically facilitate remote-assistance by connecting healthcare professional to one another. They will literally be collecting, credentialing, and connecting centers for healthcare professionals looking to assist the disaster.

The Emergency Operations Centers will be the primary nodes in the Cybercare network described above. A number of technologies – besides the network itself – will augment the commanders' abilities at the EOCs. Distributed collaboration enabled via real time audio and video is the focus of many telemedicine applications. User interfaces at the VOC level will primarily involve virtual reality technologies (VRT) and other advanced data display techniques like teleimmersion. Tele-immersion is the next logical step in remote collaboration. Users interact at great distances while perceiving that they are in the same room. Tele-immersion uses 3D environment scanning, projective and display technologies, tracking, audio technologies, robotics, haptics, and powerful networking.

Sophisticated faster-than-real-time simulations will aid in decision support by predicting possible outcomes from various actions. The simulations are similar to those used in preparation except that they must be fast enough to keep pace with the real event and flexible enough to accept situation updates from the entire response theater.

Security technologies will come into play at a number of levels. Access to command-level information will be restricted based on the position and rank of the individual person inquiring. In a virtual operations setting commanders can interact in a single command space while each individual sees different levels of information. For example, they all may be able to see virtual representation of one another, avatars; and they may all be able to see the same virtual display of the hot zone; but only certain commanders can see the virtual representations of classified resource information displayed above the virtual hot zone. Responders connecting to the network will need to be authenticated. A cyberattack into the response network that feeds commanders false information could be devastating. Although distributed, redundant sensors will be able to verify one another so that a single point of failure will not be able to disrupt the system. Finally, protecting patient medical information privacy, while limited during a disaster, is still important.

Global Positioning System (GPS) and Geographical Information System (GIS) technologies will be critical to keep track of the locations of response efforts. Locations of patients, responders, or a plume of anthrax all need to be reliably tracked and registered in relation to one another. Commanders will maintain an aerial view of the hot zone with continually updated maps of terrain, buildings, and resources. Maps should be made before the disaster and then continually updated during an event. GPS technologies also need to work within buildings and underground.

Facilities

Because local healthcare facilities – typically operating near or at capacity – will not be able to handle the sudden influx of patients new facilities will have to be established to accommodate them. The good news, as was mentioned earlier, is that bio-events typically do not require sophisticated medical interventions. Treatment primarily involves pharmaceuticals (either vaccinations or antibiotics), supportive therapy and, most importantly, isolation [7]. Assuming that containment will prevent many resources from being imported, we will build on the principle that everyone already has a private place to sleep at night.

In the event of a major bio-disaster, the government will likely ask the public the remain at home. And if the public health system can distribute basic medical supplies to them [see the Logistics section], then this probably isn't a bad place for them to be. The entire area will be isolated from the rest of the country, and individuals within the hot zone will be isolated from one another (physically). It is worth noting that this physical isolation will be augmented with cyber-communication for psychological support. Individuals, while relegated to their homes, will be able to communicate with friends and family over the internet with both video and audio communications.

The US Army Soldier Biological and Chemical Command is working on a plan for establishing emergency medical facilities called Neighborhood Emergency Help Centers (NEHCs) and Acute Care Centers (ACCs) [10]. The plan is largely based on commandeering existing facilities (schools, etc.) and converting them into healthcare facilities for triage and treatment. A variation on the idea is to convert hotels into bio-hospitals. Each patient is isolated in their own room with all of the services (bathroom, etc.) he/she needs. Each room also has its own ventilation system (perhaps a filter upgrade is required). Take all of the people currently in the hotels and convert a facility for them (like the NEHC plan as it stands now), which will require a lot less logistics than an NEHC because the guests are healthy. There are a lot more hotel beds than hospital beds in most major metropolitan areas, and bio-hotels are easier to build (and possibly more effective) than NEHCs for isolation.

Treatment

Personnel: In a containment situation, the isolated area will inevitably encounter a shortage of healthcare personnel. Historically 9 out of 10 people who approach a healthcare facility during an outbreak are "worried well" who believe they are infected but actually are not. Sorting them out from the truly infected is a major logistical hurdle but necessary to efficiently utilize resources. In addition, the truly infected must be diagnosed, categorized based on the severity of their infection, and a treatment plan must be formulated for them. All of these tasks require domain expertise that will be in short supply within the containment area. The simplest way of increasing healthcare personnel is by connecting those VA doctors reserved by NDMS around the country electronically to the disaster area. It can be as simple as a low-bandwidth, store-forward email program with a text description of the patient's medical history and a digital photo. We have used this model cheaply and effectively with minimal infrastructure to provide telemedicine in Nepal and Peru [6].

Still, these physicians will need first responders on the ground to act through. Functions of first responder include: (1) triage, (2) mass prophylaxis, (3) supportive care, and (4) community outreach. While encouraging people to remain at home rather than seeking medical attention at hospitals, treatment may come primarily in the form of door-to-door community outreach. Healthcare personnel must be outfitted with networked information technologies in order to turn them into the most efficient, effective sensors possible. Nurses going from door-to-door could have wireless handheld computers to keep track of their locations, patients treated and resources used. GPS antennae can keep track of locations, biometric sensors – like fingerprints of retinal scans – can identify patients, and bar code systems can keep track of resources. Ideally GPS and physiological sensors would be attached to the patients, but numbers and cost might make this impractical. These "Cyber-DMATs" will make the whole process of patient tracking and management more efficient. In addition to upgrading current DMATs, more DMATs need to be formed around the country to ensure an adequate number of first responders.

Logistics / Supplies

Some resources will have to enter the containment area, but none will be allowed to leave. One of the greatest resource challenges will be mass prophylaxis. Pre-incident vaccination strategies are being discussed while we write this, specifically for smallpox. While such biological countermeasures are specific to individual organisms, they are worth instituting in order to allow for a level of protection before the chaotic, time-sensitive environment of a bio-disaster. During an incident, non-infected individuals will have to be quickly vaccinated in order to prevent the spread of a disease. Alternatively antibiotics may need to be distributed throughout the population.

Information technologies, however, may be able to keep better track of the distribution of resources be they medical or otherwise. Cyber-DMATs will log the quantity and locations of physically distributed resources so that commanders maintain an accurate portrait of available resources. Robots may be useful for distributing resources in a hot zone because their numbers are easily scaled, they are expendable, and they won't spread the disease. They may even be the primary means for crossing a containment border because they can be thoroughly decontaminated without a quarantine waiting period. But at the end of the day, information technologies can only do so much. At some point, physical resources will need to be circulated, but hopefully information technologies may help to maximize those resources and avoid some of the pitfalls encountered in previous exercises.

Implementation

The Cybercare system will not be implemented overnight because of financial, logistical, political and institutional barriers. We propose a three-tiered system of implementation that will maximize protection for minimal investment and leverage existing infrastructures. The biggest change to be made is the mission change from evacuation to isolation. The major initial expense will be training.

Phase I

Phase I requires the smallest investment and little or no research effort. It is similar to a telemedicine system that we established in Nepal and Peru [6]. It is a simple, cheap form of store-forward communication that works on any computer with an internet connection and a web browser. It can be thought of as an email program with first responders in the hot zone entering medical history, physical description and a digital photo on one end and domain specialists (infectious disease physicians) on the other end.

The system might require more first responders, so investment in additional DMATs may be necessary. The domain specialists, however, will be the same one already reserved by the NDMS. The same 80,000 beds and their respective doctors that the NDMS has reserved around the country for evacuation will be electronically connected to the disaster site. But rather than being physically evacuated, the patients will be virtually evacuated. All high-level diagnosis and treatment decision will be made by the same physicians.

While real beds will have to be established at the disaster site, they will largely come in the form of people's homes. Some field hospitals – be they commandeered existing facilities or built from scratch – may have to be created for the seriously ill, and the appropriate isolation equipment will accompany them. Supplies will have to be transported to the disaster area much the same way that they are today. Command and control will remain largely unchanged except for the added responsibility of facilitating electronic connections between first responders at the disaster site and physicians around the country.

Phase I can happen today for a minimal investment and no disruption of current resources and institutions.

Phase II

Phase II of implementation focuses on outfitting the first responders to augment information gathering and patient tracking – the Cyber-DMATs. They will require the wearable hardware platform mentioned earlier to enable them to track patients in the field. Software investments include ad-hoc wireless networking and intelligent agents to ferry data around a volatile network.

Increased DMATs and medical stockpiles will expedite the movement of physical resources. Private healthcare institutions will be included in the system to harness even more remote support. Agreements will be made to commandeer public facilities to convert them into field hospitals, or equipment to make them from scratch will be stockpiled.

Training will become more important, complex and expensive. Simulation will come on the scene to help in response planning and training. Command and control will have improved communication, simple web-based coordination programs, and more data-mining and surveillance. Phase II – largely a transitional phase – will have the greatest investment in physical resources. It will improve patient tracking and pave the way for Phase III.

Phase III

Phase III is the most expensive phase of implementation and many of its component technologies require additional research. Phase III adds sophisticated networking and command and control technologies for distributed, mission C2, improved situational awareness and high-level coordination. Teleimmersion enters the picture. Sophisticated simulators will provide decision-support during an incident. The entire system will be net-centric.

Robots and sensors come into play to deliver supplies, monitor outbreaks, and track patients. Universal healthcare access should allow almost every patient to remain at home so costs of healthcare facilities and isolation equipment will actually go down. Aggressive surveillance and diagnostic capabilities in the field will be added to the list. Phase III will complete implementation of the entire Cybercare vision. Major changes will occur in the way we practice medicine.

Conclusion

No such investment in the healthcare system for a disaster that may never happen would be worthwhile unless it were dual-use and improved access to healthcare. Dual-use also helps training when parts of the system are used everyday. Such a massive federal involvement in infrastructure was best demonstrated by the Dwight D. Eisenhower System of Interstate and Defense Highways. The 160,000 miles of road cost $340 billion. It began as an infrastructure for national defense, but it ended up transforming the American economy. Similarly, Cybercare will begin as a mechanism for disaster response, but ultimately it will transform the way healthcare is provided.

The politics of implementation will be tricky. It will cut across a number of interests: public and private, state and federal. Perhaps federal standards will be executed at the state level so that states remain responsible for disaster response. Also the Joint Commission on Accreditation of Healthcare Organizations (JCAHO) could help involve the private sector.

It is important to bear in mind that the Federal Response Plan (FRP) includes 12 Emergency Support Functions (ESF) of which only one is Health and Medical Services. Most notably, food and other essential services and public works must continue to be provided to the disaster area. Clearly, the Cybercare network allows for the management of all resources, but it is worth mentioning that medical care is only part of the picture.

A terrorist attack designed to cause catastrophic levels of casualties by spreading a contagious disease or chemical or radiation illness across America must be met with a health care system prepared to respond to any and all threats and provide the surge capacity we will need in hours rather than days. A Cybercare system would protect the health of Americans, protect our economy, and, ultimately, protect our way of life. The creation of this new system will require a large-scale project that will certainly be expensive - but not as expensive as doing nothing. In addition, initial costs might be made up for in future savings. A Cybercare system would take advantage of our strengths, utilize existing resources, and could be developed rapidly if we start now.

References

[1]   Robert S. Gray, George Cybenko, David Kotz and Daniela Rus. Mobile agents: Motivations and State of the Art. Technical Report TR2000-365, Dept. of Computer Science, Dartmouth College, 2000.

[2]   ANSER. 2001. Dark Winter: Summary. Available online at:
       <http://www.homelandsecurity.org/darkwinter/index.cfm >.

[3]   Rosen, J., and C. Lucey, eds. 2001. Emerging Technologies: Recommendations for Counter-Terrorism. Hanover, N.H.: *Institute for Security Technology Studies*, Dartmouth College. Also available online at:
       < http://thayer.dartmouth.edu/~engg005/MedDisaster/ >.

[4]   Rosen, J., R. Gougelet, M. Mughal, and R. Hutchinson. 2001. Conference Report of the Medical Disaster Conference, June 13–15, 2001. Hanover, N.H.: Dartmouth College. Also available online at: *< http://thayer.dartmouth.edu/~engg005/MedDisaster/ >*.

[5]   Rosen J, Grigg E; Lanier J; McGrath S; Lillibridge S; Sargent D; Koop CE, Cybercare: The Future of Command and Control for Disaster Response. *IEEE Engineering in Medicine and Biology* 21(5): 56-68.

[6]   Joel T. Moncur, Joseph M. Rosen, MD, Shunhui Zhu, PhD, Farhad M. Limonadi. Medical Electronic Link (MEL): Providing Telemedicine on the World Wide Web. Published in Medicine Meets Virtual Reality: Global Healthcare Grid. Editors: K.S. Morgan, H.M. Hoffman, D. Stredney, S.J. Weghorst. IOS Press, Netherlands, 1997. pp 328-333. *< http://www.imel.com/MMVR%20Publication.htm >*

[7]   Henderson, Donald A., MD. "Smallpox as a Biological Weapon: Medical and Public Health Management." *JAMA*. 1999;281:2127-2137.
       < http://jama.ama-assn.org/issues/v281n22/fpdf/jst90000.pdf >

[8]   Marine Corp Doctrinal Publications – MDCP 6 Command and Control. October, 1996.
       < https://www.doctrine.usmc.mil/mcdp/html/mcdp6.htm >

[9]   Dwyer, Jim et al. Fatal Confusion: A Troubled Emergency Response; 9/11 Exposed Deadly Flaws In Rescue Plan. New York Times. July 7, 2002.
       <http://query.nytimes.com/gst/abstract.html?res=F10F16FB35550C748CDDAE0894DA404482 >

[10] Interim Planning Guide: Improving Local and State Agency Response to Terrorist Incidents Involving Biological Weapons. U.S. Army Soldier Biological and Chemical Command.
       <http://hld.sbccom.army.mil/downloads/bwirp/bwirp_interim_planning_guide.pdf >

[11] Inglesby, Thomas V., MD. "Lessons from Topoff". The Second National Symposium on Medical and Public Health Response to Bioterrorism – Speaker Transcript. Washington D.C. November 28-29, 2000. (17 Dec 2001). *<http://www.hopkins-biodefense.org/sympcast/transcripts/trans_ingl.html >*

List of Acronyms

ACC	Acute Care Center
C2	Command and Control
DMAT	Disaster Medical Assistance Team
DMW	Disruptive Mission Weapon
DOD	Department of Defense
EOC	Emergency Operations Center
ESF	Emergency Support Function
FCC	Federal Coordinating Center
FEMA	Federal Emergency Management Agency
FRP	Federal Response Plan
GIS	Geographic Information System
GPS	Global Positioning System
HHS	Department of Health and Human Services
JCAHO	Joint Commission on Accreditation of Healthcare Organizations
LAN	Local Area Network
NCW	Network-Centric Warfare
NDMS	National Disaster Medical System
NEHC	Neighborhood Emergency Help Center
VA	Department of Veterans Affairs
VOC	Virtual Operations Center
VRT	Virtual Reality Technologies
WMD	Weapons of Mass Destruction

Address for correspondence

Joseph M. Rosen, MD
Dartmouth-Hitchcock Medical Center
Department of Plastic Surgery
One Hospital Drive
Lebanon, NH 03756, USA
phone: +1 603 650 5148
fax: +1 603 650 5809
e.mail: joseph.m.rosen@hitchcock.org

A Communication-Theory Based View on Telemedical Communication

THOMAS SCHALL[1], WOLFGANG ROECKELEIN[2], MARKUS MOHR[1],
JOERG KAMPSHOFF[1], TIM LANGE[3], MICHAEL NERLICH[1]

[1] *Department of Trauma Surgery, University of Regensburg,
Franz-Josef-Strauss Allee 11, 93053 Regensburg, Germany*
[2] *Department for Management of Information Systems, University of Regensburg,
Universitaetsstrasse 31, 93053 Regensburg, Germany*
[3] *Institute for Anaesthesiology, Klinikum Osnabrueck, Osnabrueck, Germany*

Abstract: Communication theory based analysis sheds new light on the use of health telematics. This analysis of structures in electronic medical communication shows communicative structures with special features. Current and evolving telemedical applications are analyzed. The methodology of communicational theory (focusing on linguistic pragmatics) is used to compare it with its conventional counterpart.

The semiotic model, the roles of partners, the respective message and their relation are discussed. Channels, sender, addressee, and other structural roles are analyzed for different types of electronic medical communication. The communicative processes are shown as mutual, rational action towards a common goal. The types of communication/texts are analyzed in general. Furthermore the basic communicative structures of medical education via internet are presented with their special features. The analysis shows that electronic medical communication has special features compared to everyday communication:

A third participant role often is involved: the patient.

Messages often are addressed to an unspecified partner or to an unspecified partner within a group. Addressing in this case is (at least partially) role-based.

Communication and message often directly (rather than indirectly) influence actions of the participants.

Communication often is heavily regulated including legal implications like liability, and more.

The conclusion from the analysis is that the development of telemedical applications so far did not sufficiently take communicative structures into consideration. Based on these results recommendations for future developments of telemedical applications/services are given.

Introduction

The current study tries to provide an overview of a first approach to an analysis of the communicative structures of the most common telemedicine application cases, namely emergency telemedicine, teleconsultation, telehomecare, e-prescription, and internet-based health care professional education scenarios.

The following chapter introduces methods and the theoretical background relevant for the scientific methods applied in this study. Chapter 3 presents the above named cases of telemedicine and the survey of the communicative analyses of the respective cases. The last chapter describes the conclusion of the previous analyses, and tries to extract a more generic description of the communicative structures of telemedicine application as an overview. In this chapter recommendations based on the study for future developments in telemedicine are formulated as well.

Methods and Background

The methodology of semiotics and communicational theory with a clear focus on linguistic pragmatics is used to compare electronic medical communication with its conventional counterpart. The semiotic model used is based on the so-called Organon-Model [2] which has been augmented and combined with aspects of linguistic theory to provide a more complete but still useful semiotic model. The relevant subtheories of linguistic pragmatics are mainly convention theory, inference and implicature, the relevance model, and semantic role theory. The following part explains these theoretical models in more detail.

The model of communication used for this study is mainly based on semiotics and subtheories of linguistic pragmatics. The so-called Organon-Model, a semiotic model developed in [2] is central for this analysis. In conjunction with it the Co-operation Principle from [9,10] and the Principle of Relevance [21] are used for the cognitive relation between sender, addressee and message. The reference relation to perceived real world concepts is described by Reference Theory as commonly used in linguistic pragmatics [5]. Other subtheories of linguistic pragmatics like some aspects of Speech Act Theory [1,20] or interactionistic communication models [18] are not useful for this study. The current focus lies on the exchange of information and their meaning for subsequent actions, neither on actions performed with utterances (Speech Act Theory) nor on the communicative nature of any action (interactionistic theories), be it performed consciously or unconsciously. This study addresses communicative acts which are intended and which succeed, i.e. this kind of communication usually is intentional and highly relevance-oriented. Thus, the communication model consists of the basic semiotic model including reference theory, the co-operation principle, and the relevance principle.

Figure 1. Functional Semiotic Model

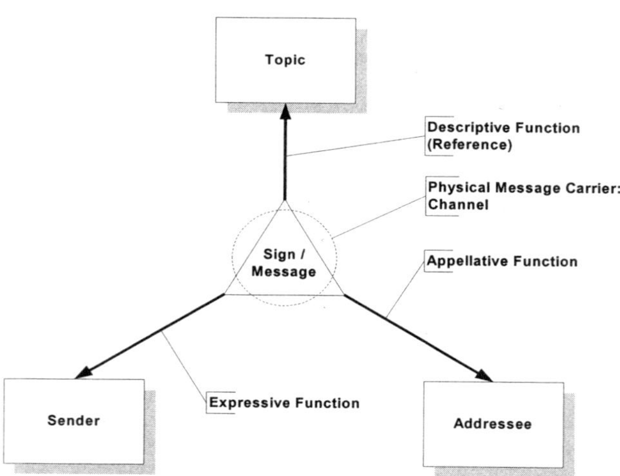

Semiotic model: For the information transmission focus of this study a code-oriented semiotic model is most appropriate. It includes the physical signal (i.e. the communication channel), and the sign/message functions towards sender (expressive), addressee (appellative), and the perceived real world concepts (descriptive, reference). This is based on the Organon-Model [2] (Figure 1). Since this study is primarily interested in communicative categories like actors, intentions, message properties, and efficiency of communication this model provides the ideal basis.

Co-operation Principle: The Co-operation Principle [9] describes communication as intentional and rational actions: 'Make your conversational contribution such as is required, at the stage at which it occurs, by the accepted purpose or direction of the talk exchange in which you are engaged.' Four conversational maxims are formulated: Quantity, Quality, Relation, and Manner. This provides an apparatus to describe especially the senders (ideal) behavior engaged in communication. Since medical communication generally is intended (even intended as maximally efficient) the Co-operation Principle provides the optimal tool for analysis.

Principle of Relevance: The addressee is the focus of the Principle of Relevance: A message is perceived if the information it provides is of (sufficient) relevance to the addressee [21]. The sender crafts the message so that it is in his opinion maximally relevant for the addressee. Thus, the sender follows the Co-operation Principle in order to achieve the required relevance for the addressee (Figure 2). This extends beyond the information of the message to the form of the message, which would mean that in medical communication any means to provide the message faster and more efficient improves the communication. Telemedical communication explicitly addresses this goal.

Figure 2. Relevance Aspects in the Functional Semiotic Model

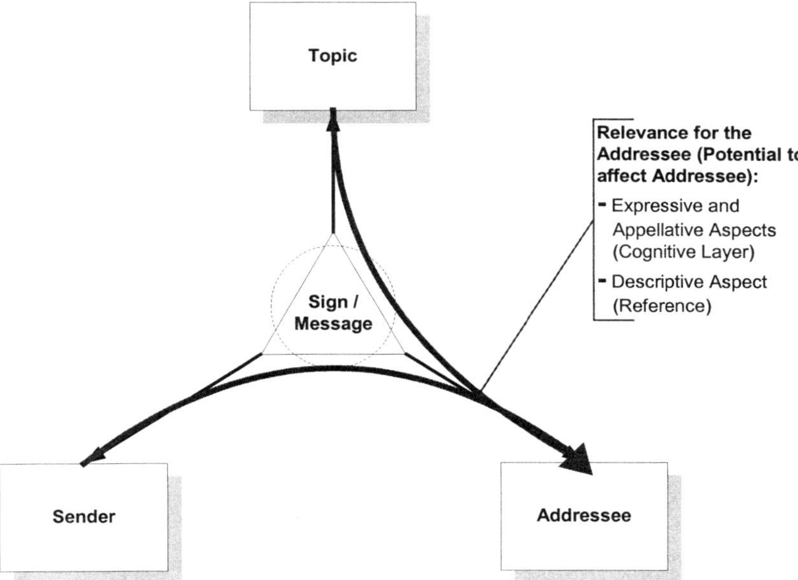

Thus, the communication model used for this study has three functional aspects which address the relation of the sign/message (which has to be realized as a physical event using a channel) to sender, addressee, and perceived real world concepts. It also addresses the cognitive principles guiding sender and addressee (Figure 3). Thus, it sufficiently provides the categories required for the current study.

Figure 3. Semiotic Model Layers

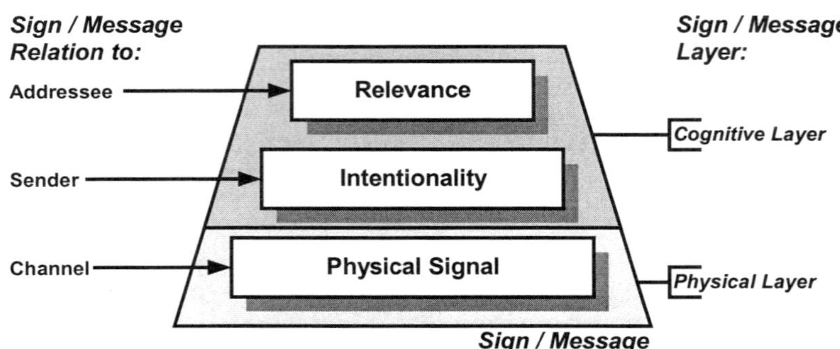

Cases of Telemedicine Communication

This chapter summarizes analyses of five of the most common cases of telemedical communication: emergency telemedicine, teleconsultation, telehomecare, e-prescription, and internet-based health care professional education. The roles of communication partners, the message structures and the relation between partners, message and perceived real world concepts are discussed. Sender, addressee, and other structural roles are identified as well as special issues like addressing a non specified addressee. Intentions and common goals, actions as consequence or prerequisite of the communicative act, and potential legal restrictions are addressed.

Emergency Telemedicine

Applications for emergency telemedicine often focus on the information flow between the emergency physician/paramedic and the clinician. Information about the case is provided by the emergency physician/paramedic for the clinician to prepare further treatment. Occasionally the clinician also is consulted about on-site intervention.

Figure 4. Emergency Telemedicine Communication Process

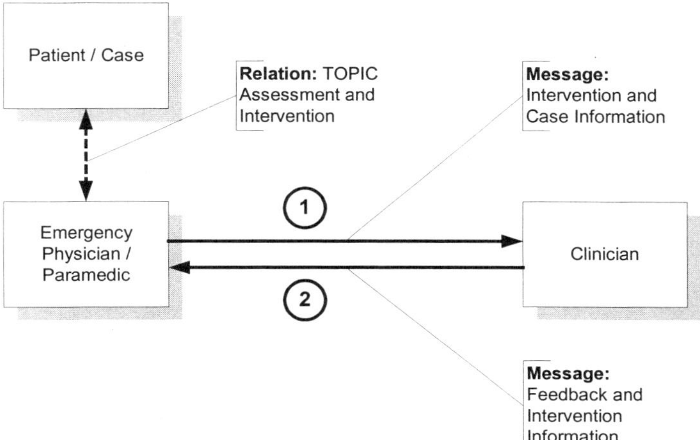

After the Emergency physician/paramedic assessed the patient/case and initiated initial intervention the following telemedical communication consists of a message about the case and intervention(s)/request for assistance to the clinician. Potentially a feedback message with intervention recommendations can follow (Figure 4). This process can be iterated if necessary.

The semiotic analysis (Figure 5) of the initial message shows that the descriptive function is fulfilled by a (partial) case description including diagnostic and treatment measures. The sender expresses the patient's need for follow-up treatment (expressive function) and requests preparation for (optimal) subsequent treatment from the clinician (appellative function).

Figure 5. Emergency Telemedicine Semiotic Structure

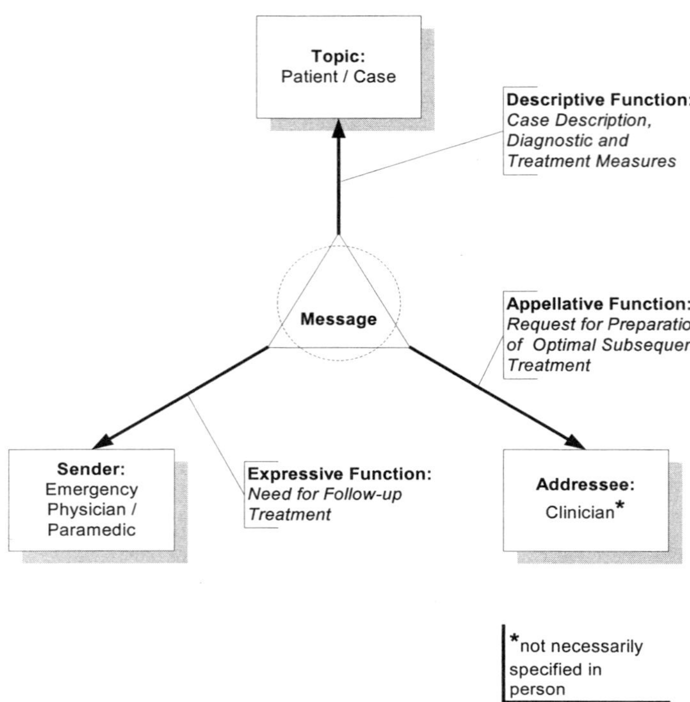

The addressee (clinician) may not be specified as an individual but is rather defined by his function (or 'role') as the emergency room physician on duty for example. The sender is (depending on the health care system) not necessarily a physician, but can also be a paramedic.

The common intention (the patient's well-being) is achieved by an action context (initial intervention and subsequent in-house treatment) that is strongly enhanced by efficient, time-critical and reliable communication processes.

Teleconsultation

Messages in the case of teleconsultation are exchanged between two health care professionals. The patient's case is introduced by the sender for assessment and recommendations on further treatment by the addressee. This subsequent treatment can often be conducted by the sender.

The health care professional conducting the treatment informs an expert about the case and previous treatment usually after assessment and treatment. The expert replies with his own assessment of the case and eventually recommendations on further treatment (Figure 6).

Figure 6. Teleconsultation Communication Process

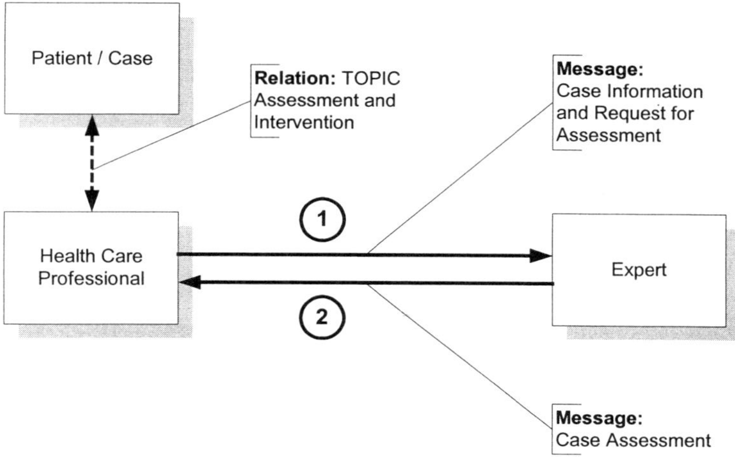

The sender's message under a semiotic perspective describes the case, ideally including anamnesis, history, diagnosis, and previous treatment (descriptive function). The expressive function shows the need for the expert's assessment of the case and further treatment. The request for assessment, recommendation (and possibly further treatment) is the appellative function of the message (Figure 7).

Figure 7. Teleconsultation Semiotic Structure

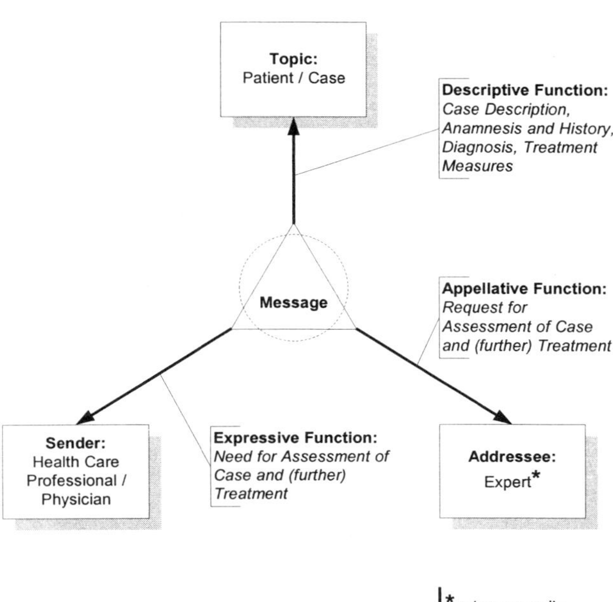

In teleconsultation the patient could theoretically become directly involved even in the communicative process between physicians (though this is rarely practiced currently). In a significant number of cases the individual addressee is unspecified but only defined by association to an institution/special field, for example. This means that addressing is role-based.

The improvement of the patient's condition, which is the common goal, is reached by getting clear about subsequent action through the communicative act.

Telehomecare

Telehomecare systems generally use a patient device to collect data either by manual entry or vital sign detection and transmit those data to a central unit which allows access to the data, eventually with analysis/digest and alarm function, by a health care professional. This information flow provides the thematic basis for the interpersonal communication process. The professional then can communicate with the patient about the monitoring results and necessary interventions. The patient can provide feedback like consent or rejection in his message (Figure 8).

Figure 8. Telehomecare Communication Process

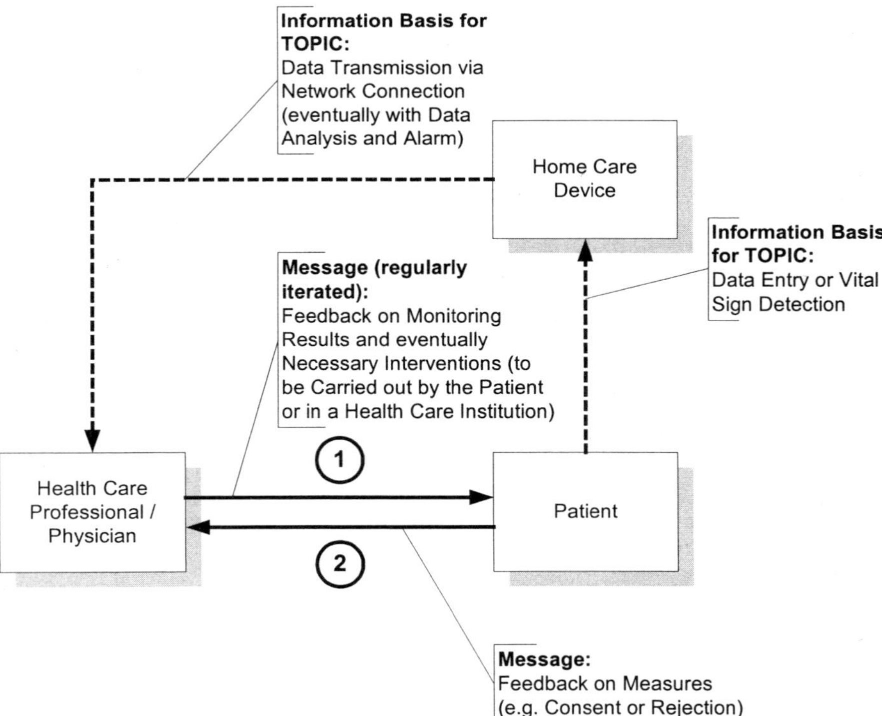

The health care professional's message contains a digest and consequences of the monitoring results, and possibly intervention measures (descriptive function). It shows his assessment of the results and maybe the need for intervention (expressive function) and provides an encouragement to proceed and/or a request to accept or carry out an intervention (appellative function) for the patient (Figure 9).

Sender and addressee are clearly specified in this communicational act. However, this is a case where the patient is directly involved as addressee, and not mainly as topic of the communication. Rather the patient (if actively entering parameters) provides actively the input which is the basis for the topic of the interpersonal communication. Thus, the common intention of the patient being well is a very personal one for (at least) one of the partners in this communication, namely the patient. This is realized by (actively or passively) providing the thematic basis for the communicational act in order to prevent intervention action or start intervention action as early as possible.

Figure 9. Telehomecare Semiotic Structure

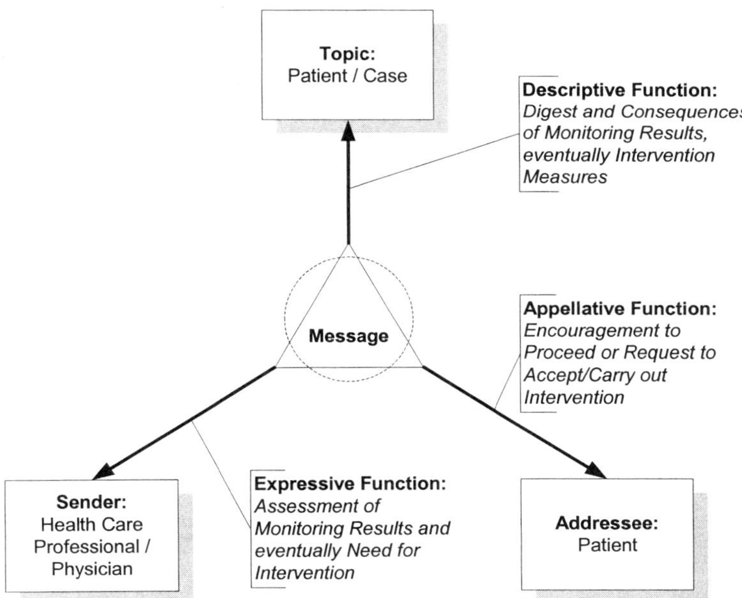

e-Prescription

In the case of (e-) Prescription the main aspect of the communicative act is that a health care professional instructs a pharmacist to perform an action: to hand out medication.

The professional's message is the request/instruction to hand out the described medication for the named patient. The patient is therefore in a topic relation to the message to the pharmacist. The action following the communicative act is thus predefined (Figure 10).

Figure 10. e-Prescription Communication Process

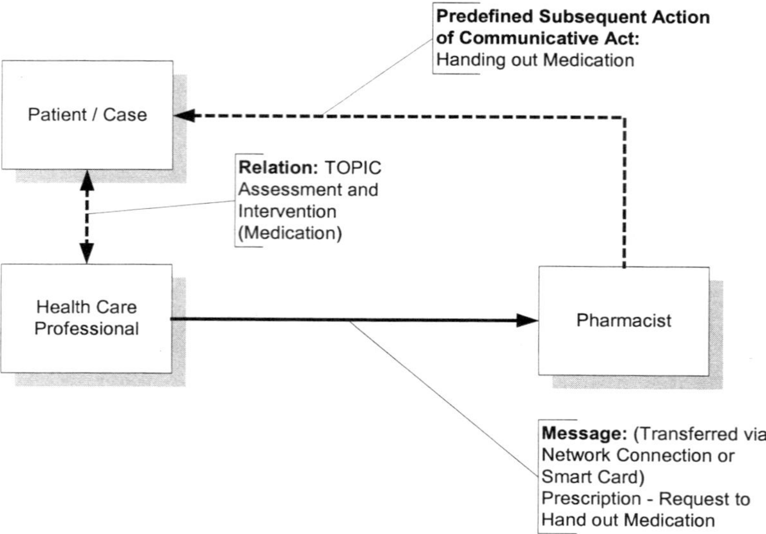

The semiotic analysis of this message (Figure 11) makes clear that the descriptive function is realized by the characterization of the required medication for the named patient. The sender asserts the patient's need for the described medication (expressive function) and requests the addressee to hand out this medication (appellative function).

Figure 11. e-Prescription Semiotic Structure

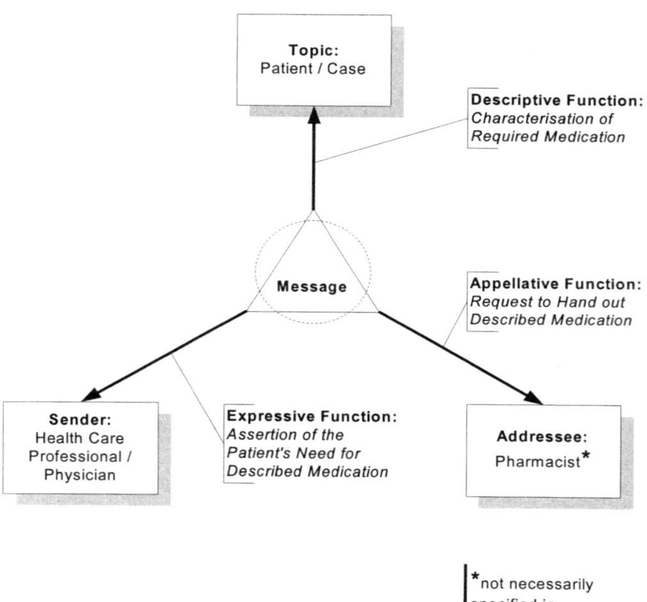

The addressee often is not specified as an individual person, but mostly role-based by the function/profession as pharmacist. In the conventional (paper-bound) case, but also in smart card based electronic scenarios the patient is not only topic but also courier, the carrier of the message.

The improvement of the patient's status (the common intention) is achieved by an action (handing out medication) that is initiated by the communicative act. The communicative act is necessary so that functional (the right medication for the right patient) and legal/administrative requirements (the patient is entitled to get the medication and the pharmacist is entitled to hand out the medication) requirements for the action can be fulfilled.

Internet-based Health Care Professional Education

Health care professional education is necessarily a communicative act since an expert shares knowledge with 'novices'. This may me mediated, in conventional cases for example by print, strongly edited as in computer based instruction systems, or highly integrated in an action context, for example in internships, but always stays communicative in nature.

There are two basic cases in internet based health care professional education:

(a)   A real discourse between an expert/lecturer and novices/audience, and
(b)   Guided case "replays" for the novices authored by an expert

In both cases this communication is usually of a one-to-many type with multiple addressees who need not necessarily receive the message at the same time.

Internet transmissions of real teaching discourses (i.e. lecture-type e-learning, also referenced as teleteaching) have primarily the message of the (medical) content the sender/lecturer intends to convey (Figure 12). The topic can be a patient's case, but also can be a digest of the expert's knowledge. The addressee's feedback message can be transferred by a different (electronic) channel like chat systems or e-mail. It can influence the sender's message only in a synchronous communication event (i.e. live transmissions), otherwise the discourse will be characterized by time delays.

Figure 12. Lecture Type e-Learning Communication Process

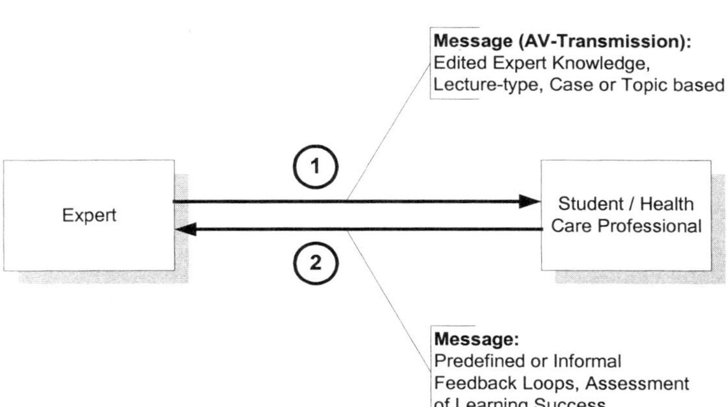

Guided case "replays" for novices by an expert are characterized by a directed stepwise communication of the message. The sender prepares the steps in an editing process to be held by an automated mediation system. This can be accessed by the addressee for a stepwise retrieval of the expert knowledge. Any feedback message by the addressee, assessment of the learning success for example, has been defined by the expert during the editing process (Figure 13).

Figure 13. CBI-Type e-Learning Communication Process

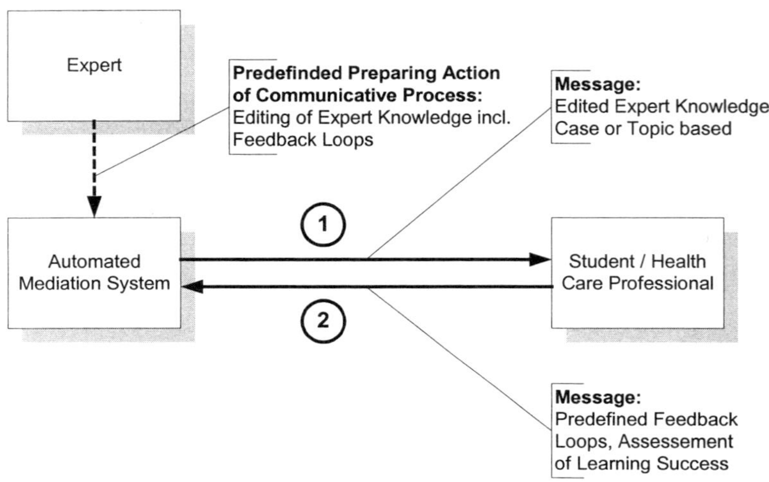

The sender's message has under a semiotic view (Figure 14) the descriptive function of conveying the edited medical knowledge, be it case or topic based. The expressive function is realized by the sender's willingness to instruct the audience (the addressees). The message's appellative function is the sender's offering of instruction of medical knowledge to the addressees.

The addressee is not clearly specified, but rather identified (actually identifies herself) by the (voluntarily of mandatory) interest in the message the sender offers. This may be limited to certain roles, i.e. professions, special fields or the like, but it is not necessarily limited. The lecture-type e-learning scenarios are modeled after conventional lecture-type learning scenarios freeing them of several spatio-temporal restrictions and imposing new technical ones. The case "replay" scenarios are rather modeled after real-life professional processes with restrictions evolving from the possibilities of technology and illustration means.

The common intention in this case is somewhat different. Primarily it is the sharing of (medical) expert knowledge in order to improve the (potential) patient's treatment in future. Thus the patient's well-being is only indirectly the intention and it is not directly related to a specific individual as can be assumed in the other cases of telemedicine communication.

Figure 14: e-Learning Semiotic Structure

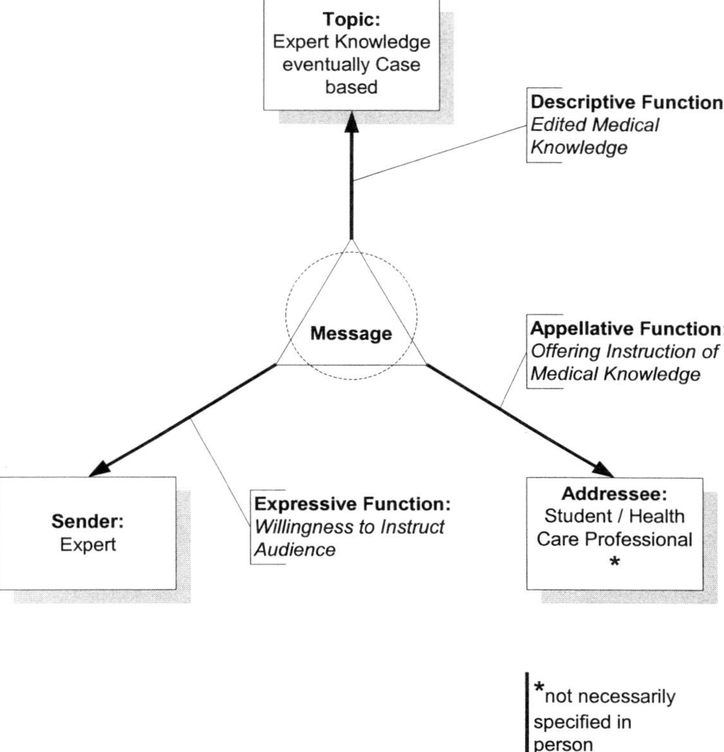

Conclusion

Communication theory opens a new view on the use of health telematics. This provides implications for the evaluation of telematics programs and projects in the health care sector. The telemedicine applications the authors have encountered so far were mostly technology-driven and thus did not include a communicative analysis at all, or they included it only implicitly or just ad hoc. A clear identification of the roles of the participants, their intentions and goals, and the structure of the message has generally not been adequate. Thus, modeling of communicative processes was almost generally ad hoc which often had negative consequences on the design of the application.

Much research has been done on the legal implications of telemedicine application. However, this has rarely been adequately modeling the actions as consequences of structured communicative acts with the mutual intention that these acts are to be performed.

In (tele-) medical communication the partners usually are two health care professionals which at least differ in their location/institution, often in special field or profession as well (Fugure 15), thus in their role. In the case of telehomecare only one partner is a health care professional, the other one is the patient. Even though all three functions generally are present, the appellative function is of central importance since the communication is intended to lead to subsequent action performed by one of the participants. The most generally formulated common goal of the participants in telemedical communication is the patient's well-being (as a last consequence this even applies to telemedical education of professionals).

Figure 15. Action Context of (Medical) Communicative Acts

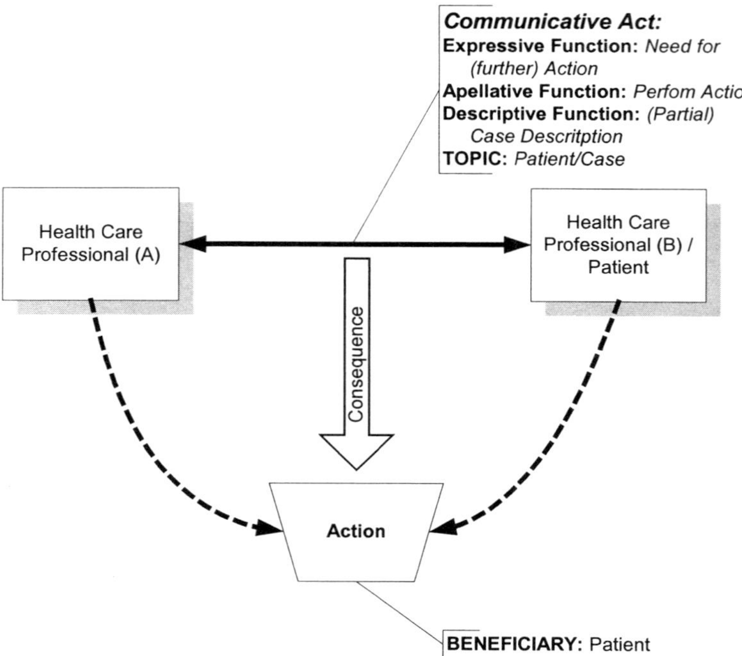

The patient usually has a defined role in this communication process, namely mostly TOPIC. However, if one wants to identify the role in the subsequent action also, it is BENEFICIARY. In future telemedicine applications this could be turned into a more active role of the patient in communication and treatment. Telemedicine can provide an efficient means to achieve this goal.

However, since the telemedical communication processes are highly structured, partially even formalized by legal/administrative regulations, they have more identifiable special features. Often the addressee is not specified in person, but rather only defined by his role, which means identifcation by the function as a health care professional, e.g. of a special field/function/profession or association to an institution. The patient often functions a courier/carrier of the message (e.g. conventional prescriptions). The communication can become more efficient if it can be multimodal (e.g. teleconsultation).

Telematic modeling of communication processes allows for several **advantages**:

- The patient needs no longer be the courier/the carrier of the message (i.e. the communication channel) in some cases.
- The communication can be richer in information content (multimodal vs. written/speech only) and often can be faster (especially compared to the written form).

- Issues like time-critical communication and high reliability of information can be resolved optimally.
- Formal requirements (legal and administrative) can be fulfilled automatically (e.g. identification of participants, documentation, formal items).
- Feedback loops can be introduced where currently are none or only insufficient ones.
- The potential for the patient to enter a more active role in the medical communication arises.

Based on these results the following **recommendations** for planning future telemedicine projects and program can be given:

- Identify roles of participants incl. the patient, become clear about special issues of the interesting communication case like addressing issues (personal addressing vs. addressing by role: profession/function/association to an institution or special field).
- Analyze the structures of the transmitted messages and find adequate and intuitive modeling for the planned electronic channel (structure of messages, type of transmission, access for communication partners, preserving the patient's rights). Try to model the communicative processes after established, working, but maybe not optimally efficient conventional communication processes.
- Name the common goal and each participant's intentions, and especially the type of action intended as following the communication process. Find out about legal restrictions and consequences and how these requirements can be met.
- Research the benefits of using the electronic channel for each participant (i.e. identify the rationale for the participants).

Thus, the authors believe that an analysis of the communicative structures of a health telematics service at the earliest possible stage can help improve the service right from the beginning and bring about the advantages of electronic communication in a more effective manner.

References

[1]   Austin, J. (1962): *How to do Things with Words*, Cambridge (Mass.): Cambridge Universtiy Press.
[2]   Bühler, K. (1934): *Sprachtheorie,* Jena (Germany): Fischer.
[3]   Cohen, P./Levesque, H. (1991): Teamwork, *Nous 25*, 487-512.
[4]   Glück, H., (ed., 1993): *Metzler Lexikon Sprache*, Stuttgart (Germany): Metzler.
[5]   Green, G. (1989): *Pragmatics and Natural Language Understanding*, Hillsdale (New Jersey): Lawrence Erlbaum.
[6]   Green, G. (1993): Rationality and Gricean Inference, Urbana (Illinois): Beckman Institute Technical Reports.
[7]   Green, G. (1994): The Structure of CONTEXT: The Representation of Pragmatic Restrictions in HPSG, *Studies in the Linguistic Sciences 24*, 215-232.
[8]   Grice, H. P. (1957): Meaning, *Philosophical Review 66*, 377-388.
[9]   Grice, H. P. (1975): Logic and Conversation, In: P. Cole (ed.): *Syntax and Semantics, vol. 3: Speech Acts* (41-58), New York: Academic Press.
[10] Grice, H. P. (1978): Further Notes on Logic and Conversation, In: P. Cole (ed.): *Syntax and Semantics, vol. 9: Pragmatics* (113-127), New York: Academic Press.
[11] Lakoff, G. (1987): *Women, Fire, and Dangerous Things*, Chicago: University of Chicago Press.
[12] Lehoux, P. et al. (1999): Theory of Use behind Telehealth Applications, In: M. Nerlich/R. Kretschmer (eds.): *The Impact of Telemedicine on Health Care Management* (29-38), Amsterdam: IOS Press.
[13] Levinson, S. (1983): *Pragmatics*, Cambridge (UK): Cambridge University Press.
[14] Nerlich, M. et al. (2002): Teleconsultation Practice Guidelines: Report from the G8 Global Health Applications Subproject 4. *Telemedicine Journal and e-Health.* 8(4):411-18

[15] Pollard/Sag I. (1984): *Head-Driven Phrase Structure Grammar*, Chicago: University of Chicago Press.

[16] Röckelein, W. et. al. (2000): E-Health Care: A Multimedia Inter-Organisational System to Support Emergency Care Process Chains, In: F. Lehner/R. Maier (eds.): *Electronic Business und Multimedia*, Wiesbaden (Germany): Deutscher Universitätsverlag, 263-288

[17] Schall, Th. (2001): New Forms of Co-operation, In: *Medical Technology in Bavaria*, Munich: Bavarian State Ministry for Economics, 12-19.

[18] Schiffrin, D. (1994): *Approaches to Discourse*, Cambridge (Mass.): Blackwell.

[19] Schug, S. (2001): *European and International Perspectives on Telematics in Healthcare*, Berlin, Akademische Verlagsgesellschaft.

[20] Searle, J. (1969): *Speech Acts*, Cambridge (UK): Cambridge University Press.

[21] Sperber, D./Wilson, D. (1986): *Relevance: Communication and Cognition*, Cambridge (Mass.): Harvard University Press.

[22] Stieglitz, S. P. (1998): Telekommunikation in der Unfallchirurgie, *Chirurg 69*, 1123-1128.

Address for correspondence

Thomas Schall, MA
Department of Trauma Surgery
University of Regensburg
93042 Regensburg, Germany
phone: +49 941 944 6805
fax: +49 941 944 6806
e.mail: thomas.schall@klinik.uni-regensburg.de

Implementation of TeleCare Services: Benefit Assessment and Organisational Models

KARL A. STROETMANN[1], VELI N. STROETMANN[1], CHRIS WESTERTEICHER[2]

[1]*empirica Institute for Communications and Technology Research, Bonn, Germany*
[2]*Philips Medizinsysteme Boeblingen GmbH, Boeblingen, Germany*

Abstract: All industrial societies are ageing. This has profound socio-economic and health sector implications. Innovative services based on Information Society Technologies (IST), like telehomecare are regarded as promising avenues to follow both to allow (national) health systems to cope with these challenges and to improve the quality of life of chronically ill and frail older citizens. The aim of the TEN-HMS project is to convincingly prove that telemonitoring of congestive heart failure (CHF) patients at home can improve medical outcome for these patients as well as their quality of life and the efficiency of healthcare delivery processes. But this will not (yet) be enough for the sustained success of such a service. Unless it takes into account the interests of the various players in the health care arena and a long-term Business Case can be proven, it will be very difficult to integrate such services into routine health care delivery processes. Before developing concrete delivery models for such a telemonitoring service, the "players" directly involved in such a service need to be identified - *customers*/patients, health services *providers*, IT services *suppliers*, and public/private insurance funds as *payers* - and their assessment perspectives considered. Then four concrete telemonitoring delivery models and their probability of success are discussed. Our analysis suggests that telemonitoring will presently only be successful if the service delivery model applied reflects national health system idiosyncrasies, takes into account established organisational boundaries and adapts to patient quality of life and health professional preferences. In the longer term, the new paradigm of seamless, patient-centred care will, however, require *new, more efficient service delivery models* integrating all aspects of the health services value chain.

Introduction

Socio-Economic and Health Sector Trends

All industrial societies are ageing. This has profound socio-economic and health sector implications [1] underlined, for example, by the dramatic increase of the *old age dependency ratio* - the ratio of the number of people aged 65 and over to the number of people between the ages of 15 to 64 - from 2000 to 2050 by, e.g., 89% in the USA and 132% in Japan (see *Table 1*) [2]:

Table 1. Development of the Old Age Dependency ratio 2000 to 2050

Year	Canada	Germany	Japan	USA
2000	0.19	0.24	0.25	0.19
2025	0.31 (63%	0.37 (54%)	0.46 (84%)	0.32 (68%)
2050	0.37 (95%)	0.49 (104%)	0.58 (132%)	0.36 (89%)

Source: Stowe, R. The Fiscal Challenge [1] and own estimates

Another factor is the steady growth in the incidence of chronic diseases, most of which predominantly affect older people and which are a major cause of them being home bound.

Table 2. Annual growth rates of various chronic diseases

Diabetes	2,5%
kidney failure/dialysis	7%
heart diseases	5%
cancer	7%

Source: Own estimates based on WHO and other publications

The implications of these two trends will be nothing but dramatic: At the same time when the financial basis, younger people in the workforce securing the economic support to provide resources for services for the older generation, deteriorates, both the relative number of those 65+ old and the absolute number of frail, chronically ill and disabled people will increase [3].

Innovative applications and new services based on Information Society Technologies (IST), like telehealth information and support services, tele homecare and telemonitoring are regarded as promising avenues to follow both to allow (national) health systems to cope with these challenges and to improve the Quality of Life of chronically ill and frail older citizens.[4,5].

This paper is based on research undertaken in the context of the European Union *Trans European Networks* project "European Home-Care Management System (TEN-HMS)". Its aim is to prove that telemonitoring of congestive heart failure (CHF) patients at home can improve medical outcome for these patients as well as their quality of life and the efficiency of healthcare processes. However, as it has turned out, this will not (yet) be enough for the sustained success of such a service. Unless it meets or takes into account the interests of the various players in the health care arena and a long-term Business Case can be proven, it will nevertheless be very difficult to integrate such services into routine health care delivery processes.

The TEN-HMS pilot implementation

The primary objective of the TEN-HMS project is to implement and evaluate a modular set of home telecare devices for chronically ill people, older/disabled citizens in need of long-term health care or patients who will benefit from constant vital data surveillance while at home. The concrete objectives are to thereby

- improve medical outcome for people suffering from chronic diseases and foster the uptake of 'best medical therapy'
- improve the quality of life of (chronically) ill people
- and to improve the efficiency (cost reduction) and continuity of healthcare processes.

In particular, the study will determine if *home monitoring* of patients with heart failure due to left ventricular systolic dysfunction at high-risk of hospital readmission can support these objectives, and if so whether home monitoring using devices to monitor weight, heart rate and rhythm, and blood pressure is superior to home monitoring by telephone contact alone.

For the study, 426 congestive heart failure (CHF) patients were selected. 12 university, teaching and regional hospitals in Germany, the Netherlands and the United Kingdom as well as local specialists and GPs are involved. By a random selection process, guided and controlled by an outside specialised institute, patients were allocated to one treatment and two control groups:

Group 1: 85 patients, follow-up according to usual clinical practice
Group 2: 173 patients, follow-up according to usual clinical practice *supplemented* by monitoring using conventional telephone contacts
Group 3: 168 patients, follow-up according to usual clinical practice *supplemented* by monitoring using conventional telephone contacts *plus* twice daily telemonitoring of vital signs

Total duration of the study was 31 months; it ended officially in July 2002, but data collection continued for some months. For methodological reasons, only afterwards detailed outcome data will become available. This experimental design - size of intervention groups, length of duration and external methodological control - make for a world-wide unique telemedicine evaluation project.

The home monitoring system is comprised of three very user-friendly electronic measuring devices (blood pressure and pulse; scale; 1-lead rhythm strip) which through standard-based (DECT) cordless communications suited to a domestic environment transmit their data to the home telephone hub. Data thus captured is automatically transmitted through secure networks to a co-operating care provider, supporting the medical staff monitoring and making decisions on treatment for the remote patients - if needed on the spot.

Assessment perspectives

Before developing concrete delivery models for such a telemonitoring service, the "players" directly involved in such a service need to be identified and their assessment perspectives considered [6]. Four main groups can be identified:

Customers/patients

For patients the medical services they receive as well as the experienced and perceived outcomes will be most important. These include an improvement or at least a stable or slower deterioration of their health situation, admissions to hospital avoided, time and travel costs saved by not having to visit a physician, or the resulting changes in the quality of life and impact on their family/household members. Subjective aspects include an improved feeling of security and of receiving better services [7]. Also important for the acceptance of such a service is the convenience and ease of use of the monitoring devices and the time and effort involved in applying them.

Such (potential) benefits will need to be confronted with the costs involved. Depending on the patient's situation, he/she will assume that his or her health insurance will cover the costs, i.e. the insurance premium will already guarantee access to such a telemonitoring service, or private payments may be needed to receive such an (optional) service.

Health service providers

For a hospital, a specialist in private office or a communal health centre offering such telehome services; their assessment will be influenced by considerations like what are the real, medical benefits for their patients, do the medical outcomes like a more stable health, fewer admissions to hospital etc. justify such a service? How can it be integrated into present work flows without disrupting exiting organisational routines, or is the necessary change worth the effort?

Other considerations concern the resulting competitive advantage vis-à-vis other health care providers in a more and more competitive, cost-consciousness environment and the costs involved in paying for an IT service provider setting up the system, leasing the measuring devices and securing its technical reliability. And, finally, what is the financial profit, are these services reimbursable, do the payments received from health insurance funds pay for the additional costs incurred, or are these fully compensated for by the internal costs saved or by the income gained from additional patients [8].

IT service providers

For them such a service must provide a clear-cut *business case*: they must be able to sustain a reliable rate of return at least equal to their present cost of capital (the rate of return at which investors are prepared to provide the company with financial funds), i.e. they must be able to recover their research and development investment, depreciate the cost of the measuring devices and infrastructure as well as their running service costs.

The IT services have to be delivered to both the patients in their home and to the medical service provider, i.e. the hospital or a local/regional community centre or physician. The most reasonable assumption at present is that a monthly service fee is charged to be paid by either the medical service provider, the patient or even the insurance fund directly. Another. less likely option would be to sell the whole system at a market price to, e.g., the care institution and leave the organisation of the technical services to them.

Payers/Insurance funds

In most health systems, medical services are paid for either by public or private health insurance and/or the tax payer, an HMO or similar organisations. Whether tele homemonitoring is an attractive option for them depends on their assessment of the benefits for their clients, cost savings expected from new ways of care, the impact on their competitive market position, and, of course, on the costs the new service involves for them.

Another assessment perspective, not explicitly introduced here, is that of *Society at large*, be it citizens, taxpayers or patients. In various instances, society will be represented by the regional/provincial or federal government, political parties, patient associations and others. To consider this would require an assessment of relevant benefits (like medical outcomes at large, quality of life, cost savings for the health system, creation of new jobs, etc.) and costs (reimbursement expenses, disruption of established health system structures and impact on important interest groups, jobs lost, laws and regulations which must be changed, etc.) at a very high level - a task we will not pursue here [9]. Also, ethical issues like universal and equal access to best medical care will not be discussed. In a very general sense, this perspective would require to achieve an optimal ratio of health outcomes/quality of life for all versus public (and private) resources allocated to health services.

In the following, in a very pragmatic approach, we present and discuss a few concrete delivery models and their probability of success. At a very general level, one can expect that new services may be successful and sustainable if all key groups concerned perceive a positive balance of benefits versus costs, or if the group with a negative balance can be compensated by another group to such an extent that it is willing to participate. However, as benefits and costs also involve such qualitative factors as power, influence, loss or gain in hierarchical position, training effort etc. such a transfer of resources from one group to another may be very difficult to realise in a concrete instance in a manner agreeable to all.

Service Delivery Models

The generic health service delivery model developed identifies the four groups already mentioned above:

- *customers*/patients
- health services *providers*
- IT services *suppliers*, and
- public/private insurance funds as *payers*.

Within this structure the customers for the telemonitoring system discussed here are heart failure patients who are being managed in an out-of-hospital settings, and who ultimately pay for the service. Normally payments will be made to insurance companies or national health systems ("Payers") in form of insurance fees or taxation. Medical services, such as reviewing the patient's status and providing medical assistance, is the responsibility of the provider (e.g. hospital, heart failure clinics or disease management organisations). Suppliers make the technical infrastructure and measurement devices available to customers and providers.

Based on our analysis and experience gained in the context of the TEN-HMS project so far, there are a number of possible configurations how the players in such a TeleCare Service Frame could group; four specific delivery models will be described.

Model A: Integration into present health system structures

The most obvious, and currently most promising model (*Model A*) is a structure in which insurance companies and national health services (payers) reimburse hospitals or medical organisations (Providers) for providing TeleCare services to heart failure patients. In turn the medical providers will purchase the TeleCare solution from the suppliers. It is depicted in *Graph 1*:

Graph 1. Delivery *Model A*: Integration of telemonitoring services into existing delivery channels

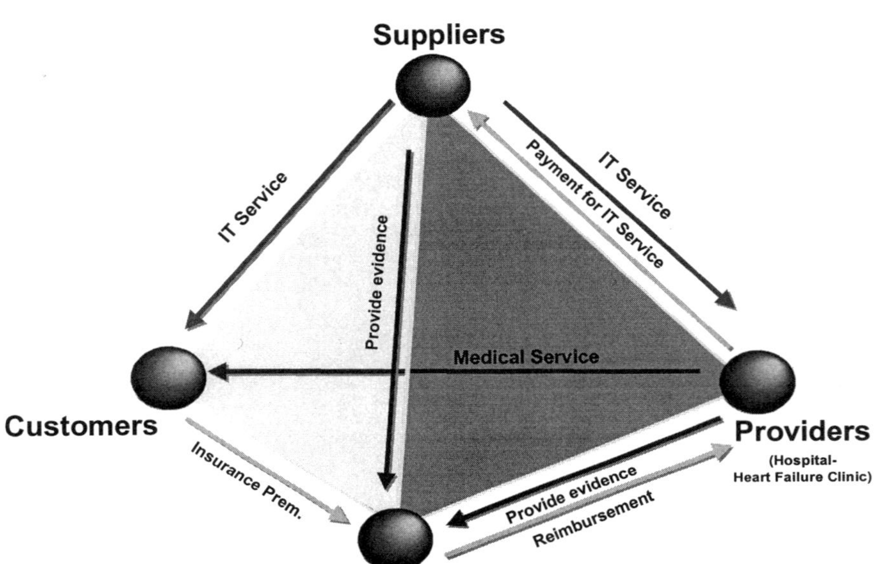

Model A assumes that the medical delivery service is provided by a health care organization (e.g. hospital, or out-of-hospital cardiology group). Normally these entities provide some form of medical service to the patients today, and view TeleCare as a logical extension of their portfolio. In most cases the Providers will be "competence centers" for a specific disease.

To foster wider-spread acceptance of such a TeleCare concept, it is of utmost importance to weave the delivery model into existing health structures. Consequently the Providers will need to network with the patient's primary care physician, thereby keeping them in the information loop. The model's medical services set-up can be best described as a hub and spoke architecture, with the Providers being the hub (Competence Centre) which offer their expertise to the spokes (the primary care physicians or out-of-hospital specialists).

Advantages of this model are:

- Patients mostly rely on their GPs as the initial point of contact when out of hospital, and can be assured their doctor is well informed.
- The TeleCare providers need the support of GP or out-of-hospital doctors to prescribe and change medications.
- Out-of-hospital doctors involved in their patient's management will view TeleCare as a benefit because it helps them to manage the patients more effectively, and not as a threat.

The IT Support Service (Suppliers) normally consists of an array of organisations such as:

- Equipment manufactures
- System integrators
- Telecommunication companies
- Device installation services

To simplify matters, in *Model A* the assumption is made that all these functions are made available through one entity, the Supplier. The Supplier is responsible for:

- providing and maintaining the entire IT infrastructure,
- installation of the measurement devices in the patient's home
- initial training of the patients and medical providers
- implementation or connection to secure networks for distributing the medical data to the care providers
- ongoing support of the TeleCare system

Payments for IT Support Services can be made in one of two ways:

- The Provider makes a one time capital investment, and purchases the entire system.
- Providers pay a license fee for each patient connected to the TeleCare system.

The inherent advantages of a license fee concept are:

- Care providers do not need to make an up-front capital investment.
- License fee payments are only driven by the number of patients connected through the system.

Within *Model A*, cash flow follows well established paths, an additional reason why this model should be relatively easy to implement. Ultimately the Customers pay insurance premiums, or are taxed for health care service. Assuming TeleCare services have been approved for reimbursement, insurance companies and health authorities will use existing structures to compensate the medical providers. The Providers in turn pay the IT Support Service a license fee, based on the number of patients utilising the system.

Because of these features, we assume that such a model will probably have the highest acceptance with both medical professionals/service providers and patients in Europe.

Model B: Combining medical service provision and IT support

One permutation of Model A is when the IT Suppliers extend their value chain to include the provision of medical services. In this case the Suppliers employ their own staff of medical professionals to monitor the patients. These combined IT support and medical service providers will either network with primary care physicians the same way hospital providers would do, or they will offer their services directly to customers. One advantage is that such a highly specialised service focusing on one or a few related chronic diseases and integrating all aspects needed to provide an efficient, reliable service can optimise work flow and delivery processes much easier - and thereby decrease costs and improve profits. On the other hand, in case other health services are needed by these patients, the "standard" health system may lack important information on the patient, refuse to co-operate with the specialised service endangering their business, and treat such patients with lower priority. - This *Model B* is depicted in *Graph 2*:

Graph 2. Delivery Model B: Combining medical service provision and IT support

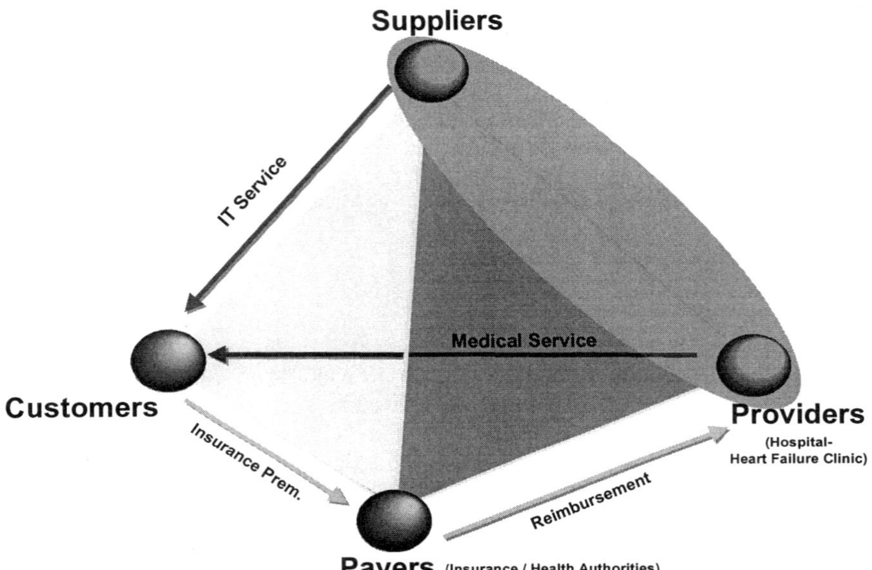

© TEN-HMS 2001

Attempts have been made to implement *Model B* e.g. in the UK, the Netherlands and Germany. To date however these providers have only had limited success in penetrating the market. The various services have not been able to penetrate the market because of patients' reluctance to accept services not delivered in the context of conventional health care systems and reimbursement issues, but also because health care providers view such offerings as a threat, and therefore are not interested in cooperating.

Model C: Managed care approach

A further TeleCare delivery model is shown in *Graph 3*. There the Payers (insurance companies) take on the role of a medical provider in addition to the classical insurance service. This structure is similar to that of, e.g., US Managed Care Organizations whereby the organisation taking on the financial risk for the patient also provides the medical service. Again, like in *Model B* due to the integration of various functions and focusing on specific medical risks an improved, more efficient service and lower costs may result.

Graph 3: Delivery Model C: Managed Care approach

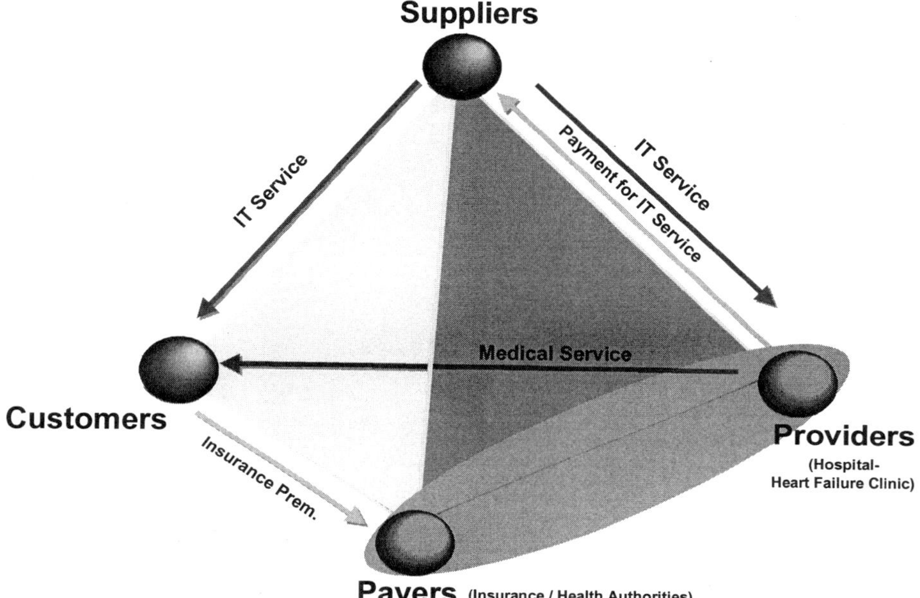

Although various insurance companies have investigated the possibility to offer TeleCare services in the context of such a model, it has currently not yet been implemented in Europe. Legal constraints and opposition by health care providers do not make this a very likely configuration for the coming years. But, e.g., in Germany *disease management* concepts to be initiated by public sickness funds are now widely discussed in health policy circles. It is foreseen to focus initially on very few, particularly costly chronic diseases, and in this context *Model C* may become an interesting option.

Model D: Private market approach

Payments by the customer, i.e. the patients or their spouse/relatives, directly to the medical and IT services providers is yet another possibility. We call this *Model D* the private market approach. No public or private insurance fund stands between the patient and the medical services. Rather, the customer shops in a free health market for the best services available and pays from his/her private pocket.

Although there is a strong and probably growing inclination by governments to have the general public pay part of their health care cost out-of-pocket, actual services financed exclusively on this basis are rare exceptions in countries with well developed national health systems. Most patients take the stand that they have paid insurance premiums and therefore expect the insurance companies to cover all their health care expenses.

Graph 4. Delivery Model D: Private market approach - direct payment by patients

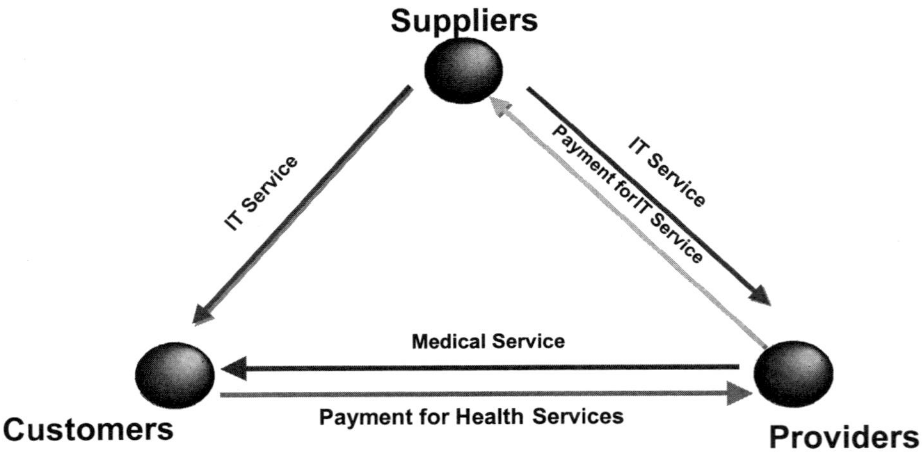

Conclusions

Demographic trends in industrial societies already have a profound impact on economic aspects like spending on pensions, health care and education. In addition, also the growing incidence of (costly) chronic diseases requires more efficient healthcare services. *Inter alia* an expansion of home care is to be expected which is not only considerably less costly than treatment in hospitals but also holds in various instances the promise to improve the quality of life of many patients and frail older people. Telehealth home monitoring is maturing and offers by now a realistic opportunity to meet some of these new health system needs.

Experience so far gained in the context of the TEN-HMS project suggests that for tele homemonitoring to expand it will not be sufficient to demonstrate - like here through a methodologically sound, randomised controlled clinical trial - the medical, patient and economic benefits of such TeleCare services. It became clear that, in addition, the interests of the various health system actors need to be taken into account when attempting to introduce new services.

The analysis of the various delivery models discussed in this paper suggests that telemonitoring will only be successful if the service delivery model applied reflects national health system idiosyncrasies, takes into account established organisational boundaries and adapts to patient quality of life and health professional preferences. Though *Model A* implies probably not the most efficient delivery work flow, it will - in the short term - be the most promising one.

In the longer term, the new paradigm of seamless, patient-centred care will, however, require *new, more efficient service delivery models* integrating all aspects of the health services value chain - from information and prevention up to long-term care.

References

[1]   Stowe, R. A New Era of Economic Frailty? - A White Paper on the Macroeconomic Impact of Population Aging. Washington, DC: Center for Strategic and International Studies - Global Aging Initiative, 2001

[2]   England, Robert S. The Fiscal Challenge of an Aging Industrial World. - A White Paper on Demographics and Medical Technology. Washington, DC: Center for Strategic and International Studies - Global Aging Initiative

[3]   Murray, CJL, and Lopez, AD. Alternative projections of mortality and disability by cause 1990-2020: Global Burden of Disease Study, in: The Lancet 1997, 349 (May 24)

[4]   Stroetmann, KA, Erkert, T. "HausTeleDienst"-- A CATV-based Interactive Video Service for Elderly People. In: Nerlich M, Kretschmar, R, eds. The Impact of Telemedicine on Health Care Management. Amsterdam: IOS Press, 1999:245-252

[5]   Balas. EA, Iakovidis, I. Distance Technologies for patient monitoring. BJM 1999;319, Nov. 13:1-3

[6]   Harris, G. Home telecare and its discontents. Telemedicine Today 1999;Aug:27-35

[7]   Stroetmann, KA, Gruetzmacher, P, Stroetmann, VN. Improving quality of life for dialysis patients through telecare. Journal of Telemedicine and Telecare 2000;6:S1:80-83

[8]   Wootton, R. Recent advances - Telemedicine. BMJ 2001;323:557-560

[9]   Stanberry, B. Telemedicine: barriers and opportunities in the 21st century. Journal of Internal Medicine 2000; 247:615-628

Address for correspondence

Dr. Karl A. Stroetmann, PhD, MBA
empirica Institute for Communications and Technology Research
Oxfordstrasse 2, 53111 Bonn, Germany
phone: +49 338 953 3000
fax: +49 228 953 3012
e.mail: karl@empirica.com

LifeGuard - Recording, Evaluation and Wireless Transmission of Medical Data

BASTIAN ARNDT, ROBERT KRANGEMANN,
MARKUS NIKLAUS, HELMUT ULRICH

*Fachhochschule Regensburg - University of Applied Sciences, Fachbereich Angewandte
Physik, Prüfeninger Strasse 58, 93049 Regensburg, Germany*

Abstract. Early diagnosis is imperative in the quest for cures for or prevention of diseases. Medical doctors nowadays can measure a multiplicity of physical determinants such as blood pressure, insulin levels, etc. The sooner this is done the sooner therapy can begin and the sooner therapy begins the greater the chances of success, no matter what the disease.

That is why self-sufficient home monitoring and emergency aid systems are becoming ever more important in medical health care.

These systems have to meet multifaceted requirements. The patient's quality of life, for example, must be maintained. Therefore the device actually worn by the patient must be light, wireless and user-friendly. Doctors must be able to operate the system easily using as little data- monitoring hardware as possible. The system must guarantee protection of privacy at all times. It should also be cost-effective and reliable. LifeGuard has been developed to meet all of these requirements.

LifeGuard is designed to record, evaluate and transmit medical data. It consists of a mobile unit containing the various individual sensors, a base station for collecting and transmitting data to a database server and a web interface for the analysis of the data (Figure 1).

Figure 1. Data flow of the complete LifeGuard system

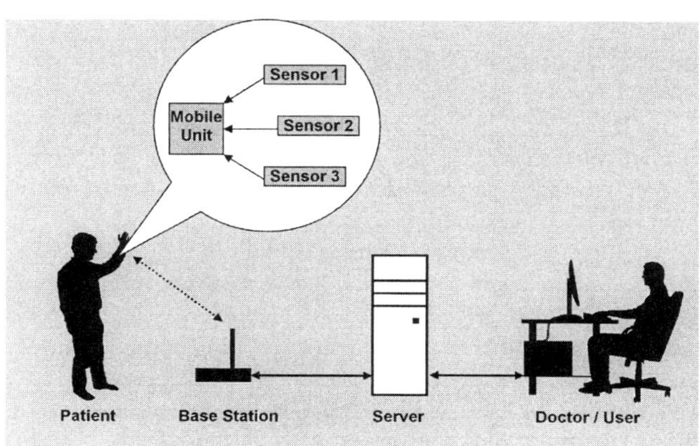

The following are the three different types of end user-:
~ The doctor who wants to monitor a patient in his home environment for a certain period of time to ascertain an exact disease pattern.
~ The patient who lives alone and needs the security of knowing support is available in an emergency.
~ The health insurance company that knows that medical therapy is usually more successful in the patients' home environment and can thus cut their costs.

Flexibility is one of the key features of the mobile unit. It is available with either just one, two or more sensors: e. g. for either temperature or pulse or temperature and pulse. The communication between the sensors is by a standard bus connector which facilitates the integration of third party sensors or the development of new sensors even without expert technical knowledge of the unit. External sensors can be connected via cable to the power supply of the mobile unit which not only reduces the cost of new sensors but also the cost of the hardware they require.

The collected data is sent to the base station at individually programmable intervals. If the mobile unit is out of range of the base station it sends a signal to the user and from that moment stores the data until transmission to the base station is possible again. The mobile unit can, in fact, collect data without sending it to its base station for a considerable time, e.g. during holidays. This feature gives the user a sense of freedom of movement.

We have aimed to make our system transparent for the user. To this purpose a liquid crystal display informs the user of each measurement and its result. Operation of the system has been kept as simple as possible. An emergency button has been implemented. When this button is activated the mobile unit sends a signal to the base station. This emergency call can be sent as soon as a problem relating to any of the measurements has been identified. The identification of the problem depends on the maximum and minimum parameters determined by the doctor who is monitoring the patient.

The mobile unit is made up of two main parts, one part contains sensors and the other the processing and monitoring unit. At present the temperature and pulse measuring functions are both integrated into the mobile unit itself, making any further external attachment of sensors to the patient unnecessary when only these two particular parameters are required. However, supplementary sensors, as we mentioned above, or other compatible sensory systems can be added externally via the bus connector. The active or passive sensors send the measured data via the simple bus system to the mobile unit where it is stored in a non-volatile memory.

The active sensors can use the power supply of the mobile unit because it is fed by the bus system in two ways-: one, with a purified 5V voltage and two, directly from the battery thus supplying a stronger current to the sensors. The bus system itself is based on the well-known I²C (Inter – IC) bus developed by Philips. This makes it very easy for third party sensor developers to adapt their own systems to fit this unit. The processing part of the mobile unit contains two Central Processing Units. This ensures that while the data from the sensor is being stored by the first CPU, the second one can access the memory, convert the data and relay it back to base by the integrated radio link. The second CPU is used for the communication with the patient. Further on there is a LCD Display where some information about the work of the unit and measured data is displayed.

The Radio Link is a bidirectional transceiver and is connected to the base station. It is possible to connect more than one mobile unit to the base station. Thanks to the bidirectional connection both, user and doctor, are able to send information back to the mobile unit where it is shown on the display. The actual radioed data transfer is safeguarded by standard codes and verified by checksums. This guarantees that approximately 99.99% of the data is undistorted on arrival, the falsified data is disposed of and a resend request is sent to the respective radio link partner.

The base station consists of a radio transmitter, a computer and a modem. The modem is not necessary if there is an existing internet connection at the patient's home. The base station is designed to support more than one mobile unit. The computer receives incoming data and stores it in a database. The computer can access the internet database in two ways - one, the regular internet connection so that the computer transmits collected data to the database server at a specific and preprogrammed time. Two, the emergency call - when the computer receives this signal, it transmits immediately directly to the database server. The connection and the transmission are always extremely encrypted to insure data protection.

The database server is always ready to receive and update data promptly. The security module of the database server is on permanent stand-by for emergency calls. When an emergency call is received all the essential data is displayed enabling the operator to initiate any rescue measures necessary. The database server has a web site which the monitor, e.g. the doctor, can use like any other internet site. The server we use to provide the monitoring interface does not require any further installation, e.g. programmes, licence files, etc in order to be accessed by personal computers both at home and at work. This is independent of the hardware or the operating system of the computer. The only software required is an internet browser such as mozilla, opera, netscape or internet explorer, one of which is usually included in every operating system. Once the doctor has been identified he can access data regarding any of his patients. The so-called webinterface facilitates not only the display of individual vital functions but also their interdependencies. Graphs and data can easily be printed out for documentation purposes. The maximum and minimum limits of the vital functions can be adjusted, should there be too many false alarms.

We realize that patient's privacy must be respected and their data protected. To ensure this we have implemented an extensive, "operator rights administration program". This allows the patient's own doctor to open a new account for another doctor whenever he requires a second opinion on any of the graphs or data he has collected. The new account only permits limited access to the data of just one specific person. This new account can then be deleted by the original account holder or an administrator.

Another way of fostering transparency is for patients to monitor their own vital functions. A messaging system which can be activated or deactivated has been implemented for closer interaction –asking and answering of questions, between user / patient and monitor / doctor.

The basic advantages of the system can be summarised as follows:
Essential for diagnosis and It facilitates essentialy a safe monitoring of high-risk patients in their own home environement. individual treatment purposes, safe because LifeGard calls for help in an emergency. The emergency call sets in motion a rapid response process, i. e. the doctor is informed, he is able to send help, information, instruction, etc. to the patient. The system can make autonomous decisions based on the data it has collected and analysed and it always reacts, even if the patient is immobile or unconscious. The patient can, in fact, also use the emergency call function for accidents not recognised by the system as emergencies such as fractures, burns etc (Figure 2).

Only ongoing observation and monitoring of patients and subsequent qualified analysis and interpretation of data enable doctors to adapt therapies to the personal habits of individual patients.

"Customised"-therapy has far more chance of success and LifeGard helps to make it possible.

Figure 2. The LifeGuard attached to a patient's arm while he is on the way
to press the emergency button

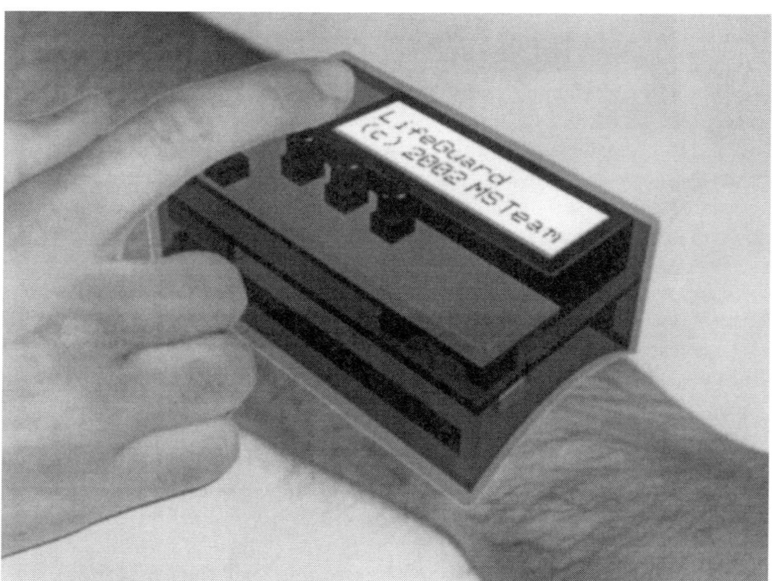

Address for correspondence

Professor Helmut Ulrich
Fachhochschule Regensburg - University of Applied Sciences
Fachbereich Angewandte Physik
Prüfeninger Strasse 58, 93049 Regensburg, Germany
phone: +49 941 943 1267
fax: +49 941 943 1426
e.mail: helmut.ulrich@mikro.fh-regensburg.de

NOAH –
A Mobile Emergency Care System

ULRICH SCHAECHINGER[1], WOLFGANG ROCKELEIN[2], ALEXANDER PERK[1],
PATRICK ASBACH[1], MICHAEL NERLICH[1]

*[1] Department of Trauma Surgery, University of Regensburg,
Franz-Josef-Strauss-Allee 11, 93053 Regensburg, Germany
[2] ZMI Center for Mobility and Information,
Universitaetsstrasse 31, 93040 Regensburg, Germany*

Abstract. The German emergency care system is a very sophisticated one. However, negative headlines like „Emergency Patient Tourism" appearing from time to time, have provoked a thorough deficit analysis which revealed two weak points: communication and documentation. The communication system presently used is a rather outdated one employing analogue voice radio between the ambulance cars/helicopters and the dispatch center and telephone communication between the dispatch center and the emergency rooms. To document the emergency case the on-scene physician is required to fill out a form. A survey showed that many of these forms are filled out incompletely and/or inconsistently or are even missing completely.

NOAH, which means „Emergency Organization and Administration Aid" („Notfall Organisations- und Arbeits-Hilfe" in German) intends to address both of these communication and documentation deficits. The on-scene physician is equipped with a mobile ruggedised PC with an internal digital radio-modem. It provides a direct, digital communication channel from the on-scene physician to the emergency physician starting from the first minutes of the treatment of the emergency patient. It also provides an easy-to-fill-out variant of the paper form mentioned above with an on-line help function and visual aids.

A typical course of events with the communication part of NOAH is as follows. The on-scene physician is alarmed via NOAH and can obtain details of the emergency during the approach. He can enter the status codes ("on the move","arrived at the emergency scene","arrived at the patient", etc.) with NOAH. During the first minutes of the treatment of the patient the physician enters a so called „First Message", which requires only 10 to 15 seconds. This message contains basic information like sex, age and the injuries of the patient. It helps the dispatch center (if the on-scene physician desires so) to make an informed recommendation where to bring the patient. This message is also forwarded to the emergency room of the destination hospital, where it can help to start appropriate preparations for the patient. When the on-scene physician has enough time, he can already bring up the documentation masks and give further information to the emergency room.

Introduction

Emergencies occur anywhere, at any location, at any time, and in various different ways - thus making any one of us susceptible.

Although the structure of the emergency care systems differ across nations, the aims in applying emergency medical services are worldwide the same:

- to save life,
- to limit damage to individual health,
- to initiate recovery procedures ensuring the best possible quality of life.

To reach these aims, the Federal Republic of Germany affords a very sophisticated emergency care system. The emergency medical services in Germany are provided by ambulance cars, vehicular emergency life support, and by helicopter - making it one of the best systems world-wide [10]. In almost all serious medical emergencies, an emergency physician on scene is alerted in addition to paramedics. The paramedics and on-scene-physicians are specially trained regarding emergency medicine and their medical equipment is highly advanced; this is why a German ambulance car or helicopter is sometimes dubbed a „Mobile Intensive Care Unit".

Due to technical and medical progress during the last few years and continued efforts to increase educational guidance for emergency physicians, emergency medical services have significantly improved. Despite good overall medical care, however, we have identified some weak points and points of non-conformance in the single phase of the rescue course which expose the patient to avoidable life-threatening situations [7,8,9]. As an example, we found that an inadequate shock treatment facilitates development of post-traumatic multiple-organ-dysfunction, which threatens the patient's life even days after an accident. On the other hand, an improperly diagnosed and treated injury can lead to a life-long disability with secondary effects in reference to social and economical problems.

Therefore, the demands placed upon any rescue system are to reduce the time that is not used for treating the patient as much as possible, and to provide the emergency physician with the means required to foster optimal care.

Whereas physicians in the hospital environment are used to work in a team and can cross-reference with others, the emergency physician on the scene is confined to make his decision without the regular diagnostic modalities. His basic knowledge has to handle specific emergencies on various specialities from gynaecology and obstetrics, paediatrics, internal medicine, surgery, and others. In case of an accident, the physician additionally has to cover managerial functions, from the initial scene analysis to timely requests for additional rescue devices, as well as the choice for the proper hospital.

This procedure must be accompanied by complete, easy to evaluate, and transparent documentation [2,3,5].

While the medical and technical progress in the field of emergency medicine has been developed (e.g., lyse-therapy on acute myocardial infarctions or new defibrillators) with considerable financial and investigative efforts, data communication and scene handling, as well as managerial functions, are comparatively underdeveloped. Primarily in the area of data communication, technical and managerial functions seem to be nearly unexplored [7,8,9].

We must therefore make an effort to optimise the information flow from the initial emergency call to the admitting hospital. Currently, communication between the emergency physician or ambulance and the dispatch-centre occurs wireless, using reserved radio frequencies (BOS-radio). Experienced communication problems are due to technical and system-related inadequacies, such as radio shadows (communication dead space), or the simultaneous use of different frequencies by the emergency physician/ambulance, fire-brigade, and police. While the use of existing direct frequencies has improved data communication regionally, this method entails considerable financial and technical efforts, and is therefore not widely used. It is the case now, as it has been before, that only one operator can communicate on any given channel at one time. The information flow also remains unchanged, dispersing unscreened and unstructured information to the operator in the dispatch-centre. This will inform the operator of the emergency physician's/ambulance location and their status, as well as additional information about other required rescue systems or special fire-brigades. This condition may foster the loss of information, or cause a delay in passing the medical condition to the admitting hospital, as experienced in the children's game "Chinese whisper" [8,9].

At the present time, it is very difficult for the on-scene rescue team to obtain quick and secure information in selecting the most advantageous hospital. This also means that the admitting hospital is not properly informed about the incoming patient.

Upon admission to the hospital, the patient should be treated carefully, effectively, and spontaneously by a pre-informed and thoroughly prepared team in the shock room. Incomplete (or lack of) incoming patient information for the admitting hospital leads to uneconomical usage of resources in cases of overestimation, and to damage to the patient in cases of underestimation.

Time loss in data communication in reference to time-sensitive situations - such as severely injured patients, intracerebral haemorrhage, myocardial infarction or poisoning - is not acceptable. These evident deficits in the intersection between rescue system and hospital have sparked headlines declaring "tourism of emergencies", when severely injured patient had to be shipped between different hospitals until one with the necessary capacity is found.

Our primary effort should therefore be concentrated on optimising the information-flow for all links within the rescue chain, starting at the emergency call and proceeding to the admitting hospital. Our goals are to specifically control available rescue-devices by means of improved communication technology, to inform the on-scene emergency physician about the availability of regional capabilities, and lastly to standardise patient reporting.

Solution-Approaches on Improving the Rescue System

Given these daily problems, the "Regensburg Emergency Services Centre" (RZR) developed an innovative communication concept for the emergency care system called "Emergency Organization and Administration Aid" (NOAH). NOAH seeks to provide a better communication link from the on-scene physician to hospitals, dispatch centres and other emergency units. Through the help of pen- or wearable-computers on-scene physicians, paramedics, dispatch centres and hospitals are in permanent contact. With NOAH, important data and information is entered in seconds and is getting forwarded in a structured way via fully digital communication channels.

Architecure of the NOAH-System

The requirements for a new communication technology encompasses the following merits:

- easy handling,
- consideration of all participants,
- integration of existing systems,
- optimised information flow during emergency missions [7], and
- avoidance of repetitive data collection [1,4].

The special requirements for an optimal pre-hospital emergency communication system are the following:

Wearable Mobile System- Hardware

- outdoor capability
- touchscreen, sensitive to pens and fingers, readable at day and night (direct sunlight / complete darkness)
- integrated smart card reader
- integrated car-printer connectivity
- integrated communication unit (speech and data)
- small size, light weight
- all kinds of interfaces (vital signs, GPS, etc.)
- continuous work without battery pack recharging for more than 8 hours and changing of battery pack within 30 seconds without loss of data
- docking station to be installed in cars and aircrafts

Various Data Input Options

- alphanumeric data (handwriting recognition / smart card)
- speech (recognition / control)
- video and still image data
- vital signs

Communication Unit

- „fire and forget" data transmission
- video / still image transmission
- bidirectional mobile speech and data communication
- wide bandwidth
- large area coverage
- maximum transmission security
- no interference with other devices

At the moment there is no system, which satisfies all these requirements, but we made some steps towards these goals.

The mobile-computer currently used is the Fujitsu Stylistic LT (see figure 1). It features a backlit VGA-compatible LCD display with a pen-based interface, an internal radio-modem for data-networks using GSM, an exchangeable internal battery providing 4 to 8 hours of operation. It is operational in a wide temperature/humidity range and has a shock-proof water-resistant design.

Figure 1. Fujitsu Stylistic LT

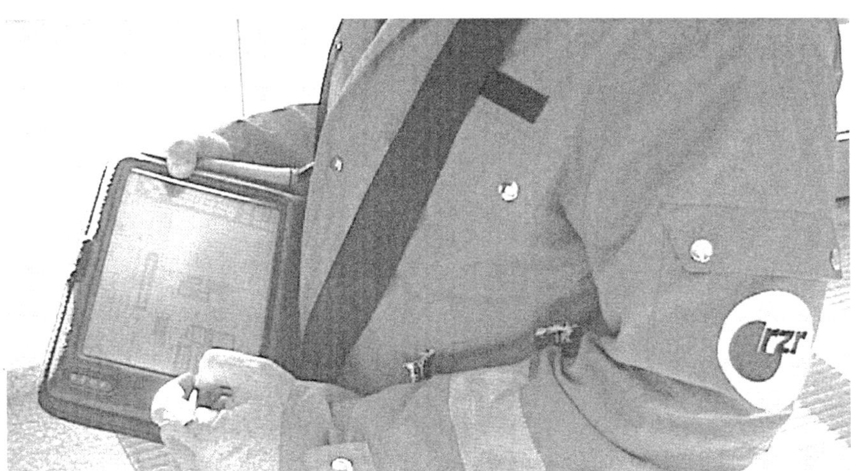

Current developments incorporate a mobile-computer in the on-scene-physicians vest, eliminating the need for an extra item to carry to the emergency scene. The NOAH-Vest employs the VIA II (see figure 2). It features a touch-sensitive Flat-Panel-Display integrated inside the vest. The other VIA II components are distributed in the vest, making the weight hardly noticeable. Another advantage of the VIA computer is that it has enough CPU power for the next updates to the NOAH-System: Voice-Control, transmission of still images from the emergency scene and GPS-based location of the on-scene physician in the dispatch centre.

Figure 2. NOAH vest with VIA II

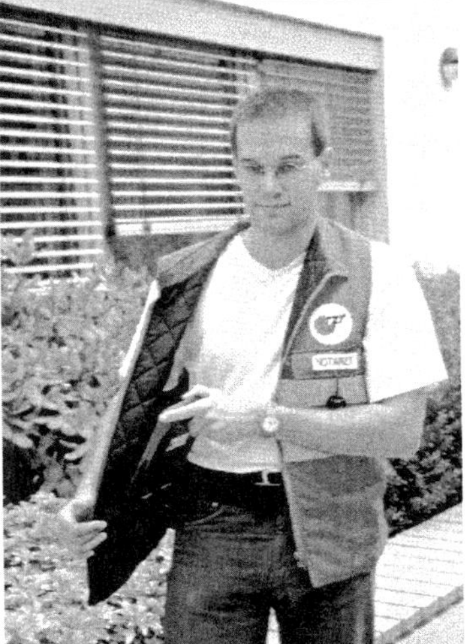
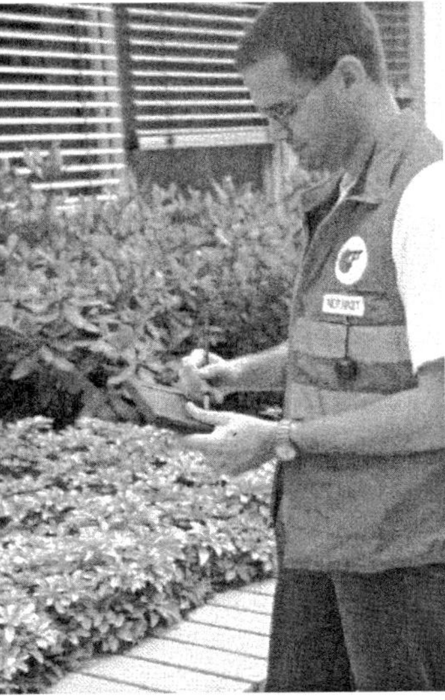

Other developments are the use of smaller mobile computers like PDAs (see figure 3) or smartphones (e.g. Compaq iPAQ or SonyEricsson P800) for the EMS-communication part of the NOAH-System.

Figure 3. NOAH communication on Compaq iPAQ

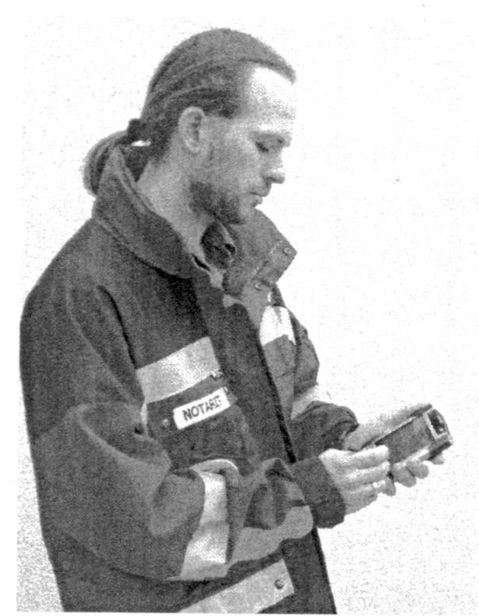

Specifically, improvement of the pre-hospital to hospital process and the documentation of emergencies is achieved by using the mobile computer loaded with an electronic version of the German Society of Intensive Care and Emergency Medicine (DIVI) standardised emergency report [2,5], and the use of mobile data transfer via the wireless data communication network GSM.

The NOAH software has been developed by an interdisciplinary team of on-scene-physicians, trauma surgeons, MIS faculty members and programmers from commercial partners.

The two methods mentioned above assist in improving the communication flow between the on-scene occurrence and the dispatch-centre. Within a few seconds, bi-directional data transfer and synchronisation with up to 1000 other participants is possible. After an emergency call reaches the dispatch centre, the dispatcher feeds the emergency instructions (e.g. the kind of emergency, location, etc.) in the dispatch center's computer system; the NOAH-communication-terminal at the dispatch centre will automatically forward this information to the mobile-computer of the alerted EMS. The respective actual EMS-status, e.g., departure or arrival at the scene, is transferred to the dispatch centre by using the notepad's shortcut EMS-status-messaging-buttons.

Upon arrival at the scene, the emergency physician feeds the notepad-computer with important information linking age, sex, emergency category, and initiated corrective action - such as intubation - and this data is sent to the dispatch-centre by a "fire and forget" method. Figure 4 shows the screen interface which is used to put the so called "first-sight information" into the computer.

Figure 4. First-sight Information Interface. Important Information is fed in the
notepad-computer upon arrival at the scene

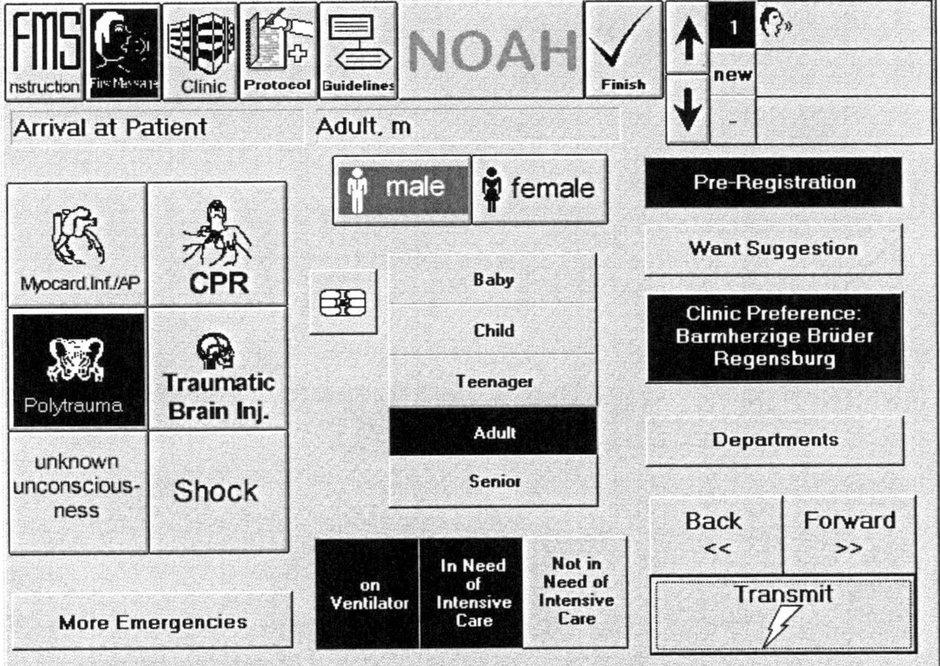

Using these data, the dispatch-centre can inform the admitting hospital in advance by
submitting significant details. Another advantage is provided through automatic
documentation recording and its selective information flow. This can be especially helpful
during disasters, when hopeless communication confusion on different radio wave channels
is experienced.

When the on-scene physician finds time he can already bring up the documentation
masks (figure 5) and give further information to the emergency room. Otherwise the on-
scene physician completes the documentation later.

Figure 5. Emergency documentation with the DIVI protocol

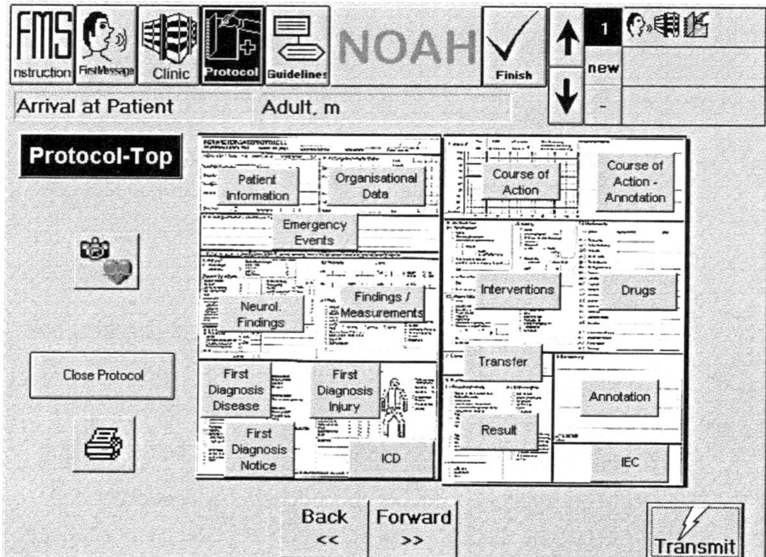

Figure 6. Entering first diagnose about injuries into the protocol

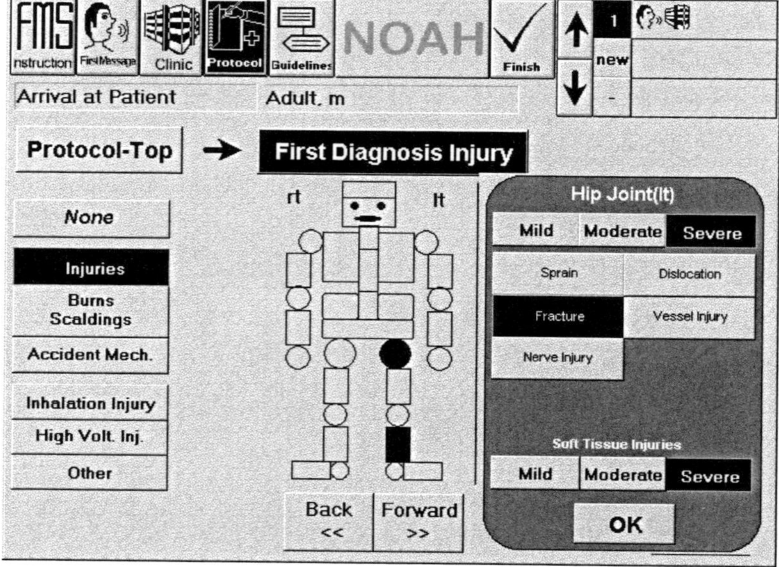

Results

The results of our studies can be summarised as follows. The usage of the NOAH system is practicable. First-sight information can be fed in less than 15 seconds, and entirely submitted within the first three minutes after arrival at the scene. This data is available at the dispatch-centre only a few seconds after its initial submission, and is available only a few minutes later at the admitting hospital as well. Practical application of this system showed a significant improvement in time (figure 7) and information processing, and was achieved through quantified information ranking (figure 8).

Figure 7. Comparison of preparation time in the admitting hopital with BOS and NOAH

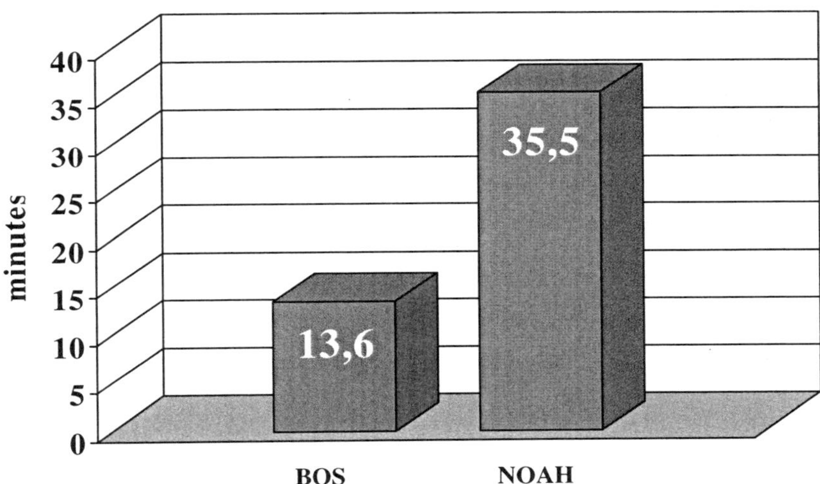

Figure 8. Information Level at the admitting hospital during emergency treatment
at the scene and patient transfer

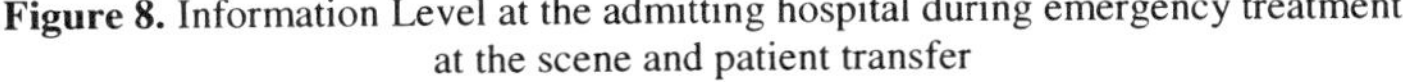

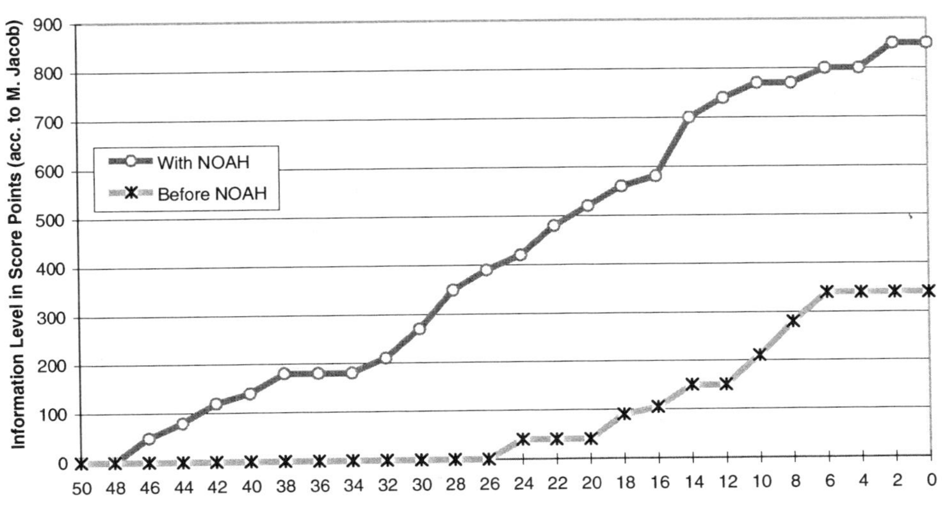

The admitting hospital was immediately and thoroughly informed of the incoming patient. There was an average time advantage of more then 20 minutes in comparison to conventional data transfer (BOS-radio), a distinct – most likely life saving – advantage.

Discussion

The NOAH-system determines a different way of information management during an emergency (figure 9). Because of the well-structured data transfer (first-sight information) to the dispatch centre only a short time after arrival on the scene, the dispatch-centre is able to pre-select and inform an admitting hospital while the emergency patient is being treated at the scene (parallel information management). Using conventional data transmission via analog BOS-radio involves serial information management, because transferring information to the dispatch-centre normally happens after finishing the initial treatment of the patient.

Figure 9. Emergency Management – Information Management

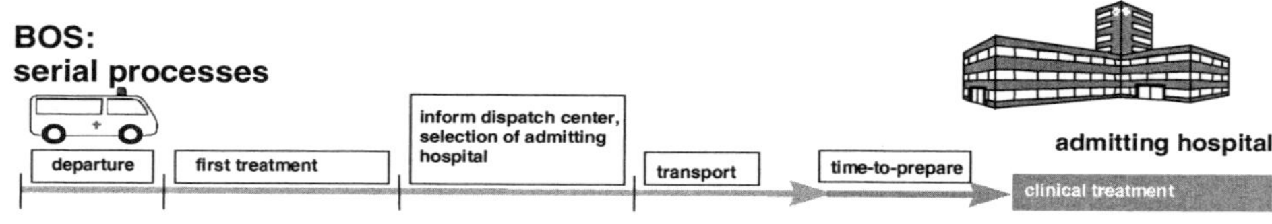

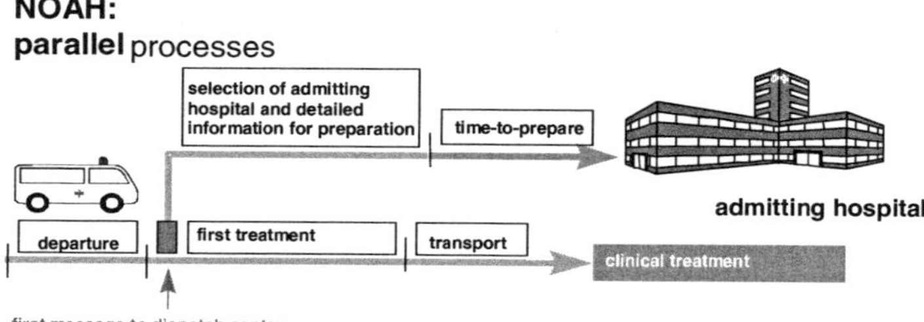

This additional time at the admitting hospital may be used to inform all needed specialists in the hospital, and to prepare for the following situations:

- preparation of the operating rooms,
- transfer of patients from the intensive care unit, and
- information transfer to on-call physicians.

High quality pre-information and high accuracy of this information reduce latency. In addition to communication facilitation and documentation, the properly programmed mobile-computer enable the flawless deposit of medical information and algorithms (figure 10) for specific emergencies (e.g., poisoning), and could lead to additional improvement in the quality of medical service provided on the scene.

Figure 10. Algorithm polytrauma treatment (in German)

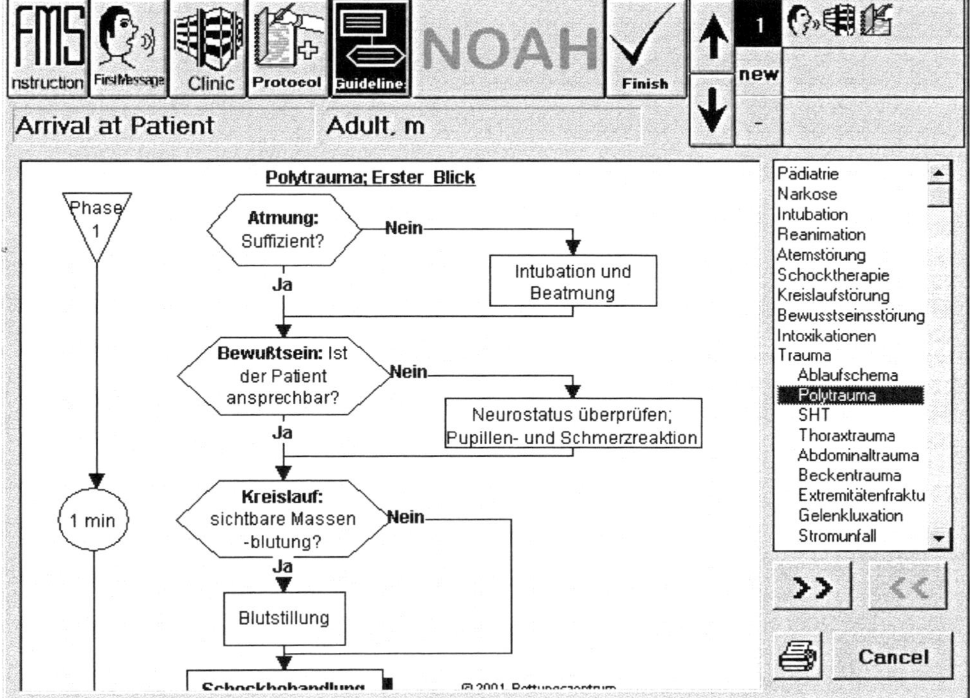

Opportunity Link of Outcome Research

This project was able to impressively demonstrate the effectiveness of the NOAH concept, which reduces the pre-clinical interval and improves flow and content of information, via:

- mobile data communication using a wearable computer with integrated modem and smart card reader (import / export of data),
- shortcut EMS-status messaging,
- „fire and forget" data transmission (First-sight Message),
- time gained by parallel information management,
- access to emergency algorithms and databases of dangerous chemicals or rare emergencies
- medical documentation

It is most important to define the medical advantage produced by this innovative application. This innovative concept shows ways to save lives, to prevent invalidity, and to improve quality of life. Statistics measuring reduction of deaths and invalidity are constantly recorded in extensive analysis projects. The NOAH-concept is currently undergoing a scientific and statistical validation programme in Eastern Bavaria. It is necessary to measure the direct, indirect and intermediate use at this point [6].

References

[1]   Collen MF. The use of documents for computer-based patient records (Editorial Commentary). Methods of Information in Medicine 1993; 32 (4): 269

[2]   DIVI. Das bundeseinheitliche Notarzteinsatzprotokoll der Deutschen Interdisziplinären Vereinigung für Intensiv- and Notfallmedizin (DIVI). Notarzt 1989; 5: 91

[3]   Donabedian A. The quality of medical care. Methods of assessing and monitoring the quality of care for research and quality assurance programs. Science 1978; 200: 856

[4]   Essin DJ, Essin CD. Computerized medical records: Software criteria for systems to document patient encounters. Critical Care Medicine 1990; 18: 100

[5]   Friedrich HJ, Messelken M. Der minimale Notarztdatensatz (MIND). Notarzt 1996,12:186

[6]   Lobley D. The economics of telemedicine. Journal of Telemedicine and Telecare 1997, 3(3):117

[7]   Maier R, Röckelein W. An Inter-Organisational System to Support Emergency Care Process Chains - The NOAH Project. Universität Regensburg, Lehrstuhl für Wirtschaftsinformatik III, 1999

[8]   Nerlich M et al. . Neue Kommunikationstechnologien in der Notfallmedizin. Rettungszentrum Regensburg, 1996

[9]   Schächinger U, Stieglitz SP, Kretschmer R, Nerlich M. Telemedizin und Telematik in der präklinischen Notfallmedizin. Notfall- und Rettungsmedizin 1999, 2(8): 468

[10] Trunkey DD. Society of Universal Surgeons. Presidential address: On the nature of things that go bang in the night. Surgery 1982; 92(2): 123-32

Address for correspondence

Ulrich Schaechinger, MD
Department of Trauma Surgery
University of Regensburg
Franz-Josef-Strauss-Allee 11
93053 Regensburg, Germany
phone +49 941 944 6805
fax   +49 941 944 6806
e-mail: ulrich.schaechinger@klinik.uni-regensburg.de

Author Index

Arndt, Bastian	143	Lange, Tim	115
Asbach, Patrick	1,147	Leong, F. Joel W.-M.	57
Bates, Joanna	51	Lillibridge, Scott	95
Baumann, Michael	83	Mc Grath, Susan	95
Benner, Thomas	15	McGee, James O'D.	57
Blobel, Bernd	25	Meier, Alexander	83
Boese, Holger	83	Mohr, Markus T.J.	73,79,115
Bruhns, Otto T.	83	Monkman, Gareth J.	43,83
Doarn, Charles R.	35	Nerlich, Michael	1,15,43,115,147
Egersdoerfer, Stefan	43,83	Niklaus, Markus	143
Ermert, Helmut	83	Perk, Alexander	147
Freimuth, Herbert	83	Raja, Kashif	83
Fuechtmeier, Bernd	43	Redl, Heinz	73
Grigg, Eliot	95	Roeckelein, Wolfgang	115,147
Haydt, Susan	51	Rosen, Joseph M.	95
Healy, Theresa	51	Schaechinger, Ulrich	15,147
Ho, Kendall	51	Schall, Thomas	115
Jackson, Andora	51	Stroetmann, Karl A.	131
Jennett, Penny	51	Stroetmann, Veli N.	131
Kampshoff, Joerg	115	Tuma, Georg	43
Kazanjian, Arminee	51	Ulrich, Helmut	143
Klein, Dagmar	83	Westerteicher, Chris	131
Koop, C. Everett	95	Woollard, Robert	51
Krangemann, Robert	143		